MINDFULNESS & YOGA SKILLS

FOR CHILDREN AND ADOLESCENTS

115 Activities for Trauma, Self-Regulation, Special Needs & Anxiety

Barbara Neiman, OTR, RYT200

Published by
PESI Publishing & Media
PESI, Inc
3839 White Ave
Eau Claire, WI 54703

Cover Design: Amy Rubenzer
Layout Design: Bookmasters
Edited By: Marietta Whittlesey

Printed in the United States of America

ISBN: 978-1-55957-012-1

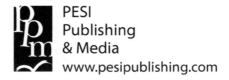

PESI
Publishing
& Media
www.pesipublishing.com

Table of Contents

Author Bio

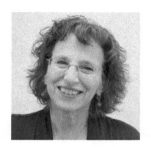

Barbara Neiman is an Integrative Occupational Therapist, Yoga Teacher 200RYT in Embodyoga®, a coach for professionals seeking a holistic practice and a National Seminar Presenter. She teaches courses on Yoga and Mindfulness around the country. She created her company, Health Discovery, in 1988, to provide services for infants through school age children. As a Certified Practitioner of Body Mind Centering® since 1989, Barbara has taught experiential hands on, movement, and meditation classes to thousands. Find her blogs on her website at www.wakeuptowhoyouare.com.

Prologue

We as humans are a connection of body systems, starting with the cells of an embryo emerging into patterns of cellular connection. As the physical structure develops, we see that support precedes movement, and the developing brain. We bundle our experiences emotionally, spiritually, anatomically and physiologically as we develop and grow, that layer into our tissues, accumulating layers of knowledge, and awareness, over- lapping, and interconnecting to become who we are. Drawing on these patterns, in the exploration of embodiment, we can find new teaching tools, new paths of learning about the body and brain. We can learn how to empower children and families with new tools and structures that they need in these complex times.

As we help children to notice a simple awareness of what they resonate with and want to move toward or away from, we are teaching a skill felt in the body that is a lifelong tool in making choices. While practicing the explorations here, we begin, unraveling, knowing, discovering, unknowing, embodying. Whether we stand still in mountain pose taking support of a yield of the skeletal system, extend our arms in a warrior 2 pose with organ awareness, or sit quietly watching our breath noticing the lungs, we have entered a new playing field. This embodied experience illuminates us as we live our daily lives, move, communicate, sense and feel to make connection with others and ourselves.

As we explore the mind of the body systems, such as the fluids, we experience the peace of meditation. Exploring basic neuro-cellular patterns of early development that underlie yoga poses, gives us information about psychological patterns. The studying of anatomy flows into a dance. The lack of support or overuse of a body system can teach us about our own somatic psychology.

Introduction

Brain Body Tools are strategies that have evolved from my own somatic, experiential study of the relationship of the mind, body, and spirit. The study grew out of my good fortune to have met and trained with teachers who paved the way for my exploration giving me a framework to live by.

The journey to understand myself and thereby help others has become my life's work. Meditation and the study of the body-mind connection dramatically impacted my skills and ability to help my clients. More profoundly, it taught me how to heal myself and gave me the wisdom to raise my child. My deepest desire is for you to do the same and to pass on tools of healing and self-discovery to those you love, work, know and live with.

I was introduced to the interconnectedness of the brain and the body at several critical junctures in my development. When I was 21, I was a modern dance student of Judith Komoreske in Palo Alto, California. Standing in front of a mirror in a garage, I had made a commitment to become a dancer. Every day, I practiced modern dance in the garage until I felt I was ready to try out for the advanced level classes.

Something powerful took place in those garage sessions. I began to connect to myself on another level. It was the beginnings of mindfulness although the word was not yet created. I stopped judging myself and approached my task patiently and open-heartedly. I redefined my identification of myself as a non-dancer to accepting myself in the present moment in my body. Instead of identifying with ideas that my body wasn't perfect, I began to ease into a space of the witness, watching myself act the role of the dancer. I explored movement principles, and worked with my muscles and brain on a deeper level. I surrendered to an emerging flow from within. To get the results I wanted, I had to live within my body and mind from that place of flow. It was shortly after this that I attended my first hatha yoga class and met my meditation teacher.

Practicing meditation has been my lifeline, helping me through junctures and crises and opening me up to an unfathomable depth of experience of my inner world. I have turned to meditation for answers through loss and deep despair. I never gave up my religion. I learned the power of going within. My experience was resolute and unwavering. No one could take it away from me, because I connected with my own self when I meditated. My family was not always supportive of my choices. Despite this, I trusted my yearning to go within for answers. I struggled with anxiety, anger and depression, but I found that as I quieted my mind, my rich wise inner self, full of light, and a sense of humor, welled up from inside to guide me. One doctor told me "you can either do medication or meditation. I chose meditation.

After a year and a half as a volunteer on a rural hospital bus working side by side with doctors, nurses and holistic practitioners, the seeds were planted for my holistic journey and passion for integrative medicine.

In 1973, when I studied occupational therapy there was little discussion about the relationship of the mind and body. Dr. Jane Ayres, a neuroscientist and occupational therapist (OT) was breaking new ground in her work on sensory integration (the study of how we take in information through our senses and process it). The psychology field still believed the brain was fixed. She believed in neural plasticity and that the brain could change itself as we now have evidence of this. Although in 2013 there were many neuroscientists and neurobiologists writing about how the brain, emotions and stress are inter-related, few existed in the 70's. Frustrated, I was looking for the course that would delve more deeply into a body-mind connection. I enrolled in The School for Body Mind Centering® founded by Bonnie Bainbridge Cohen, an OT, dancer, somatic therapist, teacher and author of *Sensing, Feeling and Action*.

I can remember my first day at the School for Body Mind Centering. One hundred of us all sat in a huge circle, each morning, and shared our life stories and reason for coming to study. It was a profound experience to enter into a community of healers, dancers, physical therapists, psychologists, and somatic educators. We studied anatomy every day by looking at a skeleton, did body work, movement, and discussion. This was the beginning of a four-summer exploration of Body Mind Centering, and later to be the central axis of my yoga study of Embodyoga®.

Bonnie's work resonated with the late Candace Pert, author of *Molecules of Emotion: The Science Behind Mind-Body Medicine*. Dr. Pert discovered that cells responded emotionally, further supporting the body-mind-spirit connection and linking science and spirituality.

Bonnie Bainbridge Cohen taught the experience of the "mind" of all the body systems and guided us through the exploration of how the different systems, skeletal, nervous, circulatory, muscular, organs and neuroendocrine could be accessed with touch, breath and movement. We also explored the developmental movement patterns and reflexes that underlie all movement and are formidable in the first year of life. Bonnie's research evolved into an exploration of embryological development. Through movement, visualization and energetic work we can explore the underlying architecture of the patterns of the brain and body and can re-pattern ourselves.

Sensing the patterns of the embryonic development experientially, we can gain new levels of understanding of the body and mind. Through this re-patterning, we explore, and free ourselves from negative patterns that may have been restrictive, or painful. During last year's Body Mind Centering Association conference, my daughter had a personal experience of internal sensing. She has never been able to swallow pills. That morning in Bonnie's workshop we were exploring through an experiential somatic exercise, the embryological development of the middle body. We were sensing the origins of the digestive track in the front of the spine. We explored this through movement, breathing and some hands-on facilitation. During class, I caught a glimpse of my daughter dancing expressively in the corner of the room, as if she had found a new level of freedom to be herself. The next day she shared that for the first time in her life, she had swallowed a pill without any difficulty. This level of somatic exploration is a powerful stepping-stone to creating change in the body's functional capacity.

Brain Body Tools has grown from this rich heritage of meditation and integrative studies. Combined with the teachings of mindfulness, Brain Body Tools will offer practitioners a way to help clients experience the connection of the mind and body.

As we learn to go within using yoga, meditation, visualization and somatic exploration, we began to witness thoughts and feelings. We enter a new playing field of sensing from the inside out and living an embodied life.

My goal is to disassemble the concepts that yoga is for physically fit people and that meditation is about stopping your thoughts. Instead, let's replace those concepts and open to the everyday applications of yoga psychology. For our children's development and our own well-being join me in exploring yoga in the world. It can help us be better parents, live more intuitive, embodied, focused and loving lives, and teach our children tools to face the world.

CHAPTER 1

The Mind Body Connection

WHY CHILDREN NEED BRAIN BODY TOOLS

Brain Body Tools are strategies for helping kids to gain confidence, relaxation and self-knowledge. In today's complex culture of stress and challenges, self-awareness that leads to self-reliance is an undeniable skill set. We must offer more to our children, a way of gaining tools for sensing, kindness for others, and self-reflection. These tools help kids by learning from "the inside" in an experiential way. In an environment, where children and adults are risking becoming disembodied by sedentary lifestyles and screens, yoga and mindfulness is an anchor back to physical and mental health. When we explore using the breath and movement we learn about sensation and how information comes to us through both the body and mind. These tools can be used with all children and can help those with trauma, special needs, sensory and attention issues. Brain Body Tools can help children who are stressed by grounding them through the senses and somatically. As clinicians, we want to better position young people with ways to stay present in their bodies, in the moment.

THE IPAD VERSUS SENSORY LEARNING: THERE IS ROOM FOR BOTH

Children, parents and teachers are spending more time with screens (phones, computers, iPads®). A concern is the danger that kids get less conversation with adults and one another. There is less physical activity, embodied learning and sensory experiences. Children literally are replacing feeling objects in their hands, with touching them on a screen. For example a child was shaking a cup with dice for the Yahtzee® game. Trying to be helpful, the principal asked the child if he would like the app for the game on his iPad. My goal was for the child to move his arm and hand as he shook the container. I wanted him to feel the smooth texture, temperature of the dice and to hear the sound the dice made as they hit the table. I was using the sensation from shaking the jar for proprioceptive input. By simply using the app, these goals would be lost in the experience; all the sensory motor experiential learning removed. For children who are educationally deprived, the many virtues of the iPad don't need to be mentioned here. As we all know many amazing ways that the iPad is contributing to learning. What are of great concern are the somatic learning experiences that may be lost, the eye contact and personal interaction with other students and adults that the iPad is replacing within family life. Screens may be depriving children of feeling, touching, and sensory experiences. It concerns me that in some families children are no longer expected to have a dinner table conversation when eating in a restaurant. Instead, they are placated with an iPad or phone. Are we denying our children relational and conversational experiences? How does a generation of children that cannot tolerate downtime affect society? The impact of too early exposure to screens on very young children's brains is yet to be determined.

BRIDGING YOGA AND TECHNOLOGY

Despite these caveats, I have observed that the smart board is a dynamic tool for therapy and can evoke engaged responses from even very autistic and handicapped kids. Smart boards are large white boards that operate as a touch screen device, they project and display websites, images and videos. They provide classrooms with opportunities for interactive learning. I have worked in classes with autistic children using the smart board to engage with a yoga DVD. My concern is that often the student may be sedentary at the smart board while using the apps and programs. As therapists, we are excited to see students respond to an app. Yet, from a movement perspective, I often wonder if we might be asking too little from them. Yoga offers us options. A weight-bearing, ambulatory student before touching the board with a wand may be able, with support, to do the triangle pose and then cross midline to touch the screen. A weight bearing, partially ambulatory adolescent may be encouraged to stand with support in mountain pose or attempt tree pose before touching the screen. Including yoga adaptations and support with the smart board may offer therapists and students, new options for body-mind exploration.

How Yoga Can Enhance Sensory Regulation

Many therapists utilize sensory modalities to help children and adolescents learn to regulate their feelings and behaviors. The sensory processing issues affect the child's ability to adjust to transitions, textures, noise, etc. Children may be sensory seekers, under-responders or over-responders. Yoga can be used to stimulate, calm and reduce anxiety.

Over-Responders, Under-Responders or Sensory Seekers Can Benefit

Under-responders who need alerting benefit when tuning in somatically to a balance pose. Their lack of interest in socializing and noticing when they have injured themselves is typical of these children. A partner yoga pose is excellent for an under-responder with its social interaction. They can be taught to notice, recognize and accept sensation. The over-responsive child may have too many reactions to transitions, textures and feelings. They are often seen as sensory defensive. These children react strongly to odors and noise. The over-responsive child might enjoy the restorative poses where there is not too much stimulus. The sensory seeking child who is in constant search for more sensation through movement and the environment and has difficulty sitting still will benefit from the both the physical breaks to the day that yoga brings and the added movement to the body.

Yoga can affect a shift in the nervous system from the activating sympathetic to the calming parasympathetic branch. This can help children to better modulate sensation and tolerate it as they become more comfortable, relaxed and calmer. There are postures that can help the over-responder, the under-responder and the sensory seeker.

Yoga offers a threefold experience, slow movements that release tension and are calming for the mind, *Pranayama* breathing that is regulating by tapping into the parasympathetic nervous system and asanas (postures) that are focusing. Performing deep breathing allows a gentle somatic experience of the body. When a child feels safe in the space, and the pace of the session is comfortable, he or she can feel relaxed.

When a therapist teaches a child or client to breathe deeply and feel into the body, the child can slowly allow themselves to experience sensation. Once the trust is established, the client can have a somatic experience while combining the yoga posture and the breath. Whether you are an over-responder or an under-responder, the different varieties of postures, breath and hand mudras (a hand position that activates the nerve endings on the fingertips to promote relaxation) can be used to create a treatment plan. This can be incorporated into a sensory diet that is appropriate for that child and for the entire family.

Yoga With Children in Groups and Individual Sessions

As an OT, I have been doing individual yoga sessions in schools and in groups for over 30 years. I have found that children love doing yoga. They enjoy being on the floor, the moving and the relaxation. Sometimes, they might be resistant at certain ages, but as long as I kept my voice gentle and made it fun, the children would engage. In the exercises and activities described in this section, we will explore using yoga for toddlers, preschoolers and sensory classroom sessions.

The Embodied Exploration

Embodyoga and Body Mind Centering study and apply knowledge of the body systems such as the skeletal, muscular, nervous, organs, circulatory, and endocrine to movement. Underlying yoga postures are body systems, movement patterns and the body-mind connection. Bonnie Bainbridge Cohen explains the relationship of organs and the initiation of movement in this way: "Organ support precedes initiation of breath, which precedes movement."

For example, the heart organ can support in a back bend. In the sphinx pose, the chest and heart are opening, and the upper extremities are weight bearing into the hands and forearms in a push pattern. The heart and hands connect in the pose of the sphinx. This can then help us to understand the emotional tone of certain yoga postures as a "heart opener" when the front body and chest is expanded through a pose. In this small backbend, the heart is opened and expanded and the arms are yielding and pushing into the earth. Backbends, which are energizing and open the thoracic area, seem to help depression. Yoga has been noted to lower cortisol, a stress hormone.

In *Wisdom of the Body Moving* (1995), Linda Hartley describes this energetic connection:

> *The energy of the heart is expressed through the hands and also provides support for them as they move in space. The energy of the organs needs to be allowed to reach through the limbs and out into space; to do this we need to go through another system, such as bones, muscles, blood or nerves. The heart also supports the upper body, spine and head when weight is taken on the forearms and hands as in the "sphinx" posture. The weight of the heart is transferred through the bones of the hands and its energy radiates out through the hands, as the hands push into the floor, this impulse levers back into the heart to give support to the spine at this level. This also helps lift the head. Gravity is not just a downward force but also supports upward and works with us to support us(p.186).*

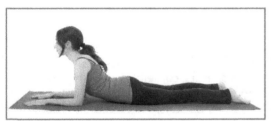

Sphinx Pose

Sphinx Pose

Donna Farhi, author of *Yoga, Mind, Body and Spirit* explains simply:

"With the emphasis on opening the heart, lungs, and chest, backbends exhilarate, bringing a sense of lightness and vitality that wards off even the most tenacious lethargy or depression. Almost all of our daily activities bend the body forward."

Think how children sit at desks, bending over writing, reading, eating, and at computers.

ACTIVITIES FOR OPENING THE HEART

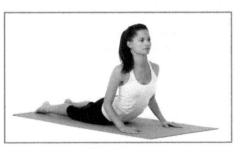

Cobra Pose

Opening the Front Body: The Cobra

- Tap the sternum, clavicle (collar bone) and feel the side and bottom ribs
- Become aware of the heart and lungs inside the bone structure
- Practice light backbends
- Cat and Cow warm-up
- Sphinx (connect the hands to the heart)
- Cobra (experience the heart, lungs open)
- Bridge pose (connect head to tail)
- Counterbalance with Child's pose
- Sponge pose (*Savasana*)

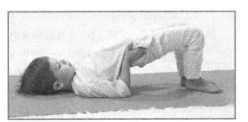

Bridge Pose

The Heart Flashlight: Illuminate your World Guided Imagery

- Come into full expression of Sphinx or Cobra
- Focus by inhaling and exhaling with the equal breath. With each inhale count to 4 for the length of the breath and count to 4 for the exhale. Do two rounds of 4 counts on the inhale and exhale.
- Imagine a beam of green light spraying love from the heart
- See the light illuminating everything and everyone
- Greet the world with a big hello from your heart
- If there is a situation that is creating stress or anger for you, imagine sending the green heart ray there like a gentle rain or a fire hose depending on what is needed.

Adaptations: This exercise can be done in these other optional positions as in the illustration below of reclining crossed leg pose (*Supta Baddha Konasana*)

- Seated in a chair as Cow pose with hands behind head
- Mountain *(Tadasana)* Sponge pose *(supine)*
- Partner pose: Back-to-back breathing seated, arms linked in slight back bend
- Reclining crossed leg pose
- Comfortable seated, supine or side-lie position

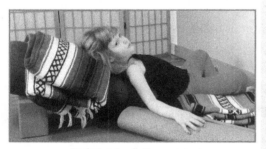

Reclining Angle Pose

Reclining Angle Pose (*Supta Baddha Konasana*)

This position is very restful for a sensory corner. It is an easy and comfortable way to have the body supported and to feel immediate rest and rejuvenation. Use a wedge, bolsters, blankets, pillows or bean chair to raise the back slightly off the ground, at an angle of about 45 degrees or what is optimal for the client. The body can be in a half-sit and half-lie position with the sacrum at the edge of the bolster on the mat as the torso is positioned leaning on the bolster with head support. Position the feet together as in a cobbler pose, soles touching with knees bent and supported with pillows under the thighs as the legs splay downward. An eye pillow can also add supportive rest. This pose is suggested without the use of a belt for a school or therapeutic session.

MUDRAS FOR MOOD MANAGEMENT

The ancient yoga teachers and Dr. Jean Ayres, originator of sensory integration, recognized the tactile sense for its significance in mood management. Both acknowledged that the fingertips have many significant nerve endings. The ancient yoga teachers understood that positioning the hands and the fingers could impact moods for energizing or calming. These hand positions are called mudras in yoga. In their book, *Mudras for Healing and Transformation*: Joseph and Lillian Le Page, founders of Integrative Yoga Therapy, state: "Mudras are a hidden treasure that open us to our own innate resources for healing at all levels of our being. "Mudra, which means seal, is a way of directing energy flow in the body and creating relaxation.

The mudras can be combined with breathing and with guided meditation, or you can start the yoga session and end with a hand mudra for focus. I found that doing a hand mudra would bring an immediate shift of awareness and direction of attention into the body.

ACTIVITIES AND MUDRAS FOR MOOD MANAGEMENT

The Tulip: Lotus (*Padma*) Mudra

I find this mudra to have an immediate calming effect. It is related to the throat area of the body and is for communication and relaxation. It can be combined with deep breathing. I teach this to teachers to do with students when the activity level of the room is getting too high. When I practice it, I immediately drop into a still place of calm. I have taught this mudra to special needs teens and they became very relaxed using it in combination with guided imagery.

How to position the hands for The Tulip

1. Position the hands near the heart and throat area.

2. Place the hands together palms touching and fingers pointing upward.

3. Spread the fingers of all the middle fingers.

4. Maintain the pinky and the thumbs connected.

5. Press the base of the wrists together and open the middle fingers outward as if the hands were the shape of a "tulip" or a bowl.

6. Sit in a comfortable posture.

7. Gently yield your feet into the floor if you are in a chair.

8. Combine with deep breathing

9. Sit quietly and embody the calm from this mudra.

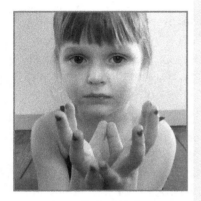

Lotus (Padma) Mudra

YOGA AND CHILDREN WITH SENSORY PROCESSING ISSUES

As an OT working with kids with sensory issues, keeping postures simple and allowing students to become acclimated over time has worked best for me. I have included certain postures that have worked for particular children on my caseload. I have set up sequences with postures that can calm, focus and aid in self-regulation. Alerting poses are also listed here. You may have different results; this is a framework to work from in your exploration.

These sequences are suggested for interacting with a sensory subsection, but it is important to be flexible and responsive in the moment as this is an exploratory approach. The poses were selected to provide weight bearing, deep breathing, relaxation, balance, core strength, range of motion, opening of the heart and alerting as needed. You may find favorite poses that work for your clients that are not mentioned here, as these are a few suggestions.

ACTIVITIES FOR CHILDREN WITH SENSORY ISSUES

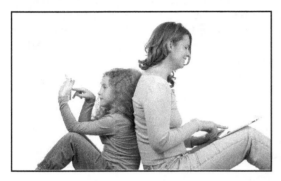

Back-to-Back Partner Breathing

Back-to-Back Partner Breathing

This back-to-back breathing activity incorporates a body mind centering principle of distinguishing the right and left lobes of the lungs, the layering of the body systems and the awareness of the cells.

- Sit comfortably with your partner on the floor with legs crossed back to back. If you are unable to sit on the floor, you can sit sideways on chairs with the chair backs facing your right sides.

- Quietly start to notice your own breathing and notice the breathing of your partner.

- Notice the air passing through your lungs with a cellular awareness of your layers of skin, muscle, bone, organ, blood, and nerves.

- Notice the cells that make up all these systems.

- Notice the three lobes of the lungs on the right side and the two lobes on the left side. Notice there is a distinction between each side.

- Notice your back muscles and the structure of your bones and those of your partner.

- Notice how it feels to breathe through all the body's layers and the lobes.

- Notice when you're breathing in sync with your partner's breathing.

Adaptation: Positioning Multi-handicapped Students for Partner Breathing

Adapt this pose for a multi-handicapped child or adolescent by setting up in a side lie position. Placing the student's back to your front body, allow the child to lean into you (yield). Or, you can sit and lean back into a bean bag chair, secured ball or a wall with the student's back body positioned to lean back into the therapist's front body, sitting between the therapist's legs. If the student can't be positioned like this, place the student's hand on your stomach, sternum or clavicle and allow the student to experience your breathing pattern. The student can also watch a tissue, toy, paper or ball as it moves on their belly while breathing. If these techniques aren't doable, refer to the accommodations by the equal breath activity. Once positioned, proceed with the directions above for the partner breathing.

- Simple Instructions for three-part breath and partner breath

  - Inhale and watch your breath within go up through the three chambers (lower part of the abdominal area, the thoracic region or mid-section of the chest and the area under the clavicle or shoulders and upper chest region. Follow this with an exhale down through the same three chambers.

  - Repeat the inhale and exhale 10 times.

  - Sense the breathing of your partner and imagine the breath going through the skin, muscle, bones, circulatory system, organs and lungs.

  - Notice what happens to your breathing sitting with your partner.

Back-to-Back Partner Breathing in chairs

- If there isn't time or accommodation for students to sit on the floor, they can sit sideways on chairs for partner breathing. The students can do back-to-back breathing on chairs sitting sideways.

- Instruct the children to arrange the chairs, with the chair backs facing their right sides so they can sit back to back.

- For chairs with desk attached, their backs would be positioned where they enter the seat, and then their legs are extended through the other side.

Hatha Yoga, *Vinyasa* and Restorative Yoga for Sensory Issues

Hatha yoga is the name given to effort to do the physical poses. *Ha* also mean sun and *tha* means moon and it means the unity of the sun and moon or the universe.

The definition of *Vinyasa* is linking body movement with breath to form a continuous flow. *Vinyasa* quiets the mind by activating the parasympathetic nervous system. *Vinyasa* can utilize poses to alert or calm. Just as the hatha yoga postures in this workbook are helpful for self-regulation, the restorative poses bring a deeper relaxation. Restorative yoga poses are done lying down or sitting and use props. They are called restorative because of the deep relaxation and rejuvenation that comes from doing this active relaxation.

The three following sensory seekers' sequences combine active poses, vibration breath (Humming Bee), guided imagery, relaxation and meditation (See chapters 3 and 7). The poses can be interchanged and have a relaxation component, Sponge or Do-Nothing-Doll pose at the end.

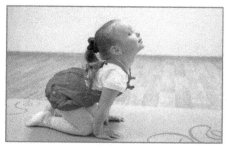

Cat Pose

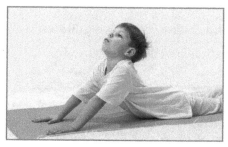

Cow Pose

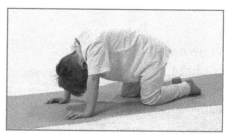

Upward Dog

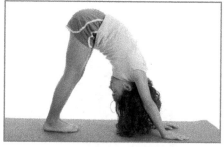

Downward Dog Pose

Hatha Yoga and Sensory Seeking Children

Series A: Active Poses

- Moving warm-ups and seated side bends
- Cat
- Cow
- One Leg One Arm balance
- Upward Dog
- Downward Dog
- Triangle
- Tree
- Bridge
- Child pose
- Three-part Breath
- Sponge

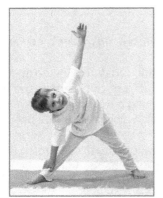

Triangle Pose

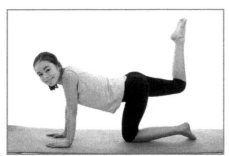

Three-Legged Kick Pose

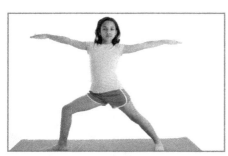

Warrior 2 Pose

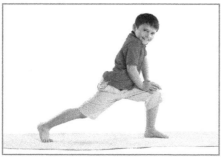

Deep Lunge Pose

Series B: Active Poses

- Forward Fold (*Uttanasana*)
- Triangle
- Tree pose
- Plank
- Bridge
- Back and Forth Rolling
- Three-part Breath and guided imagery and meditation
- Sponge pose

Series C: Vibration Breathing, Warm ups and Restorative Yoga

- Humming Bee breath
- Moving warm-ups
- Upward Dog
- Down Dog
- Mountain
- Warrior
- Plank
- Guided imagery and meditation with legs on wall

End with Sponge pose and eye pillow, or a restorative pose such as legs up on the wall or Child pose over a big pillow

Hatha Yoga and Over-Responsive Children

- Guided somatizations (Three- part Breath)
- Forward Bend
- Downward Facing Dog
- Three- legged Kick
- Cat and Cow
- Plank
- Sphinx
- Mountain Pose
- Warrior 2
- Deep Lunge
- Tree

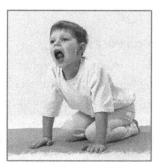

Lion Pose

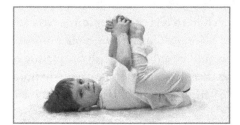

Happy Baby

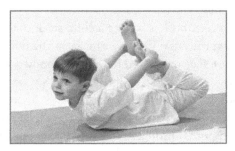

Bow Pose

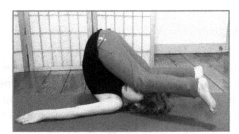

Plow Pose

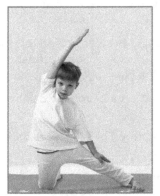

Knee Balance Pose

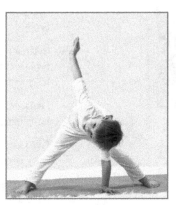

Forward Wide Angle

- Lion
- Restorative Legs on Wall
- Equal breath with long exhale (inhale 4, hold 4, exhale 4)
- End with Sponge pose

Hatha Yoga and Under-Responsive Children
Shorten the series to the client's tolerance

- Humming Bee breath
- Supine moving warm-ups
- Happy Baby
- Hip openers seated to cobblers
- Bow
- Plow
- Rocking movements in supine, knees to chest
- Cobra
- Bridge
- Table
- Knee balance poses
- Mountain
- Triangle
- Forward wide angle and twist extend arm up
- Partner Pull Pose
- End with Sponge pose
- Short story and guided imagery

TOOLS FOR CALMING THE NERVOUS SYSTEM

Sensory Regulation Solutions, Restorative Yoga Poses

Clinicians look for activities to help children to self-calm and self-regulate. A child who is over-responsive and reacts too easily to stimuli would benefit from using the restorative poses as a self-calming activity. They can easily be added to a therapist's toolbox. When a child is feeling angry, anxious, or traumatized, a basic restorative pose can feel very safe and comforting. Positioning the body with props under the knees and neck feels extremely restful and self-contained and can include an eye pillow. For children with sensory, trauma, balance, sleep, and regulatory issues, relaxing in a basic restorative pose allows the body to yield into the earth and feels secure.

Sensory Corners: Partitioned Environments with Less Stimulation

A sensory corner is a quiet and secluded area in a classroom or home for a child to relax and minimize extra stimulation. It can be portioned off with furniture, a small tent, a screen or a specified place. Adding a few simple props in a sensory corner in a classroom would allow for restorative poses. A sensory corner would be enhanced with the picture of the pose posted on the wall. The restorative poses support the body in all planes, so there is no tension in having to hold the body up. When the limbs, head, neck and chest are supported so a person isn't striving to hold against gravity, an effortless state can occur.

Simple Restorative Poses for the Classroom, Home or Therapy Session

A simple pose that needs no equipment is "legs up against the wall" where you lie supine on the mat and place your legs at 90 degrees on the wall. Another simple pose that can be done in a classroom is having a child stack their fists one on the other and simply put their head on their fists to rest while seated at the desk. Or they can sit on the floor and put the legs through the chair legs and rest the head on the chair seat either on fists or stacked hands. The body doesn't have to work at all in a supported forward seated posture with a pillow for the torso, called supported child's pose. Have the child sit with the knees folded under them and ask them to bend forward from the hips. Lay the entire torso and head over a large cushion that allows them to rest. The child can also sit on the floor with legs extended and place a therapy ball between the legs while leaning forward over a ball for a restful seated pose. Or on a mat, Child's pose can be used as a restful pose, where the child kneels and bends forward laying the torso onto the mat. The head rests down on the hands or the hands can come to the side of the body. These restful poses allow for a deep rejuvenation.

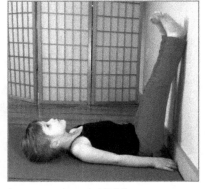

Legs on Wall Pose

Legs Up on the Wall

In a restorative pose "legs up against the wall" place the child supine on the mat and place his legs at 90 degrees on the wall or on a chair. To get into this pose, simply have the child put one side of the hips up against the wall, and then swing the legs up onto the wall as they lie down on their back. Position the buttocks near the wall according to comfort level.

- Instruct the children to sit next to a wall and position the right hip next to the wall, with legs extended straight alongside the wall.

- Instruct the child to swing the legs up and rest the legs on the wall while lying down in supine. Some students may prefer a folded blanket under the hips.

- Legs can be also placed on a beanbag chair, wedge, chair, or stabilized ball.

- Give children a blanket, towel or sweater as body temperature may drop.

- Adolescents with a large torso may need neck support with a rolled towel. The neck should not be hyper-extended backward. Adjust as needed with props to support and raise the neck for proper alignment.

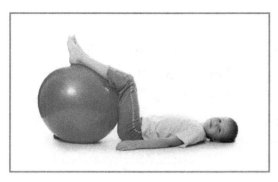

Legs on a Ball Pose

Adapted Equipment Version: Legs on a ball

Legs on the wall can be adapted for special populations or situations by using a chair, stabilized ball, a low bench, wedge or bolster depending on the size of the child. In this adaptation, the legs are flexed at an angle of 90 or more degrees and positioned on a ball. This works well in a sensory corner, therapy session or added to a sensory diet regimen for a home program.

The Belly Elevator (Practicing the Three-part Breath)

- Place a toy, tissue, paper, ball or animal on the student's belly.
- Begin the deep three-part breathing.
- Notice the breath coming into the belly.
- Watch how the inhale makes the toy go up with the abdomen extending.
- Watch how the exhale makes the toy go down with the abdomen contracting.
- See the three-part breath activity in Chapter 5.

Resting on Stacked Fists on Desk

- Have the child stack his fists one on top of the other at the desk
- Put the head on the fists to rest while seated at the desk
- Do the equal or counting breath (count 4 for the inhale and exhale)

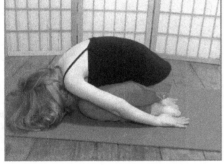

Child's Pose

Child's Pose

A restful pose to do after doing active poses, is Child's pose. This can be an alternative for Sponge pose in a sensory corner for a child who doesn't want to lie down.

- Start in a quadruped position
- Sit back onto the heels, lower the chest to the thighs
- Extend the arms forward, chin to the chest or place arms along your sides
- Lean over equipment such as pillows, blankets, towel rolls, or bolsters for a supported Child's pose.
- For an adapted, restorative or seated pose for children who don't want to lie down, extend the legs out in front of the body with a V and place a pillow, bolster, or ball between the legs placed in front of the body. Instruct the child to lean forward onto the supports used and hug their arms around it while resting.

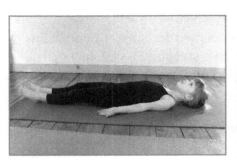

Sponge Pose

Sponge Pose

- Have the child lie down on his or her back on a mat or rug to rest
- Place arms at sides and put the palms face up on the floor
- It is also referred to as the Do-Nothing-Doll pose
- While resting, the body temperature drops
- Offer a blanket, towel, or jacket to keep warm
- For a seated pose, lean over a pillow or bolster placed in front

TIPS AND TAKE AWAYS

1. Watch for somatic and physiological responses
2. Be flexible. If a child wants to stop, respect that
3. Be creative. Alternatives to Sponge pose are Child's pose, legs on the wall, leaning over a ball, hugging a bean bag chair or seated with head on desk
4. Avoid forcing or overly focusing on any child
5. Only use praise
6. In a one to one session, you can play quiet music to create a calm ambiance and repeat a simple sequence for 10-20 minutes and rest in Sponge pose.
7. Enjoy yourself and be happy with small results. It is ok if the children don't want to do all the poses. The children gain from being in the presence of your calm state and "breathing into stillness." Have fun and keep at it.

Yoga can be offered to students from early childhood to adolescence for calming, alerting, mood management, and deep rest for rejuvenation. By building a sensory corner at home or school, implementing breathing into a sensory diet program, or helping a student have more movement breaks in class or with smart board yoga adaptations, we are offering students a connection to the mind and body. Exploring with a flexible mind, a sense of humor and enjoyment is key for the teacher/therapist. As we relax into the poses, we open emotionally to a somatic exploration. We begin understanding the application of Brain Body Tools.

CHAPTER 2

Yoga for the Classroom: Pre-school, therapy sessions and with the profoundly handicapped

A simple *Vinyasa* warm up sequence can assist a parent, teacher or therapist when providing a yoga intervention for children. A yoga intervention is a hatha or restorative yoga pose, movement series, breathing exercise or guided imagery that offers a break or empowers the students and caregiver to meet their goals. These brain body tools facilitate the child to energize, focus, regulate emotionally and calm. These activities can take as little as 2 minutes or up to 15 minutes depending on the time allotted.

Seated *Vinyasa* Sequence for a classroom

Sitting in a chair, begin to breathe in the three-part breath (See Chapter 5). Reaching both arms overhead take an inhale. Exhale as you move the arms down again. Repeat this five times.

Seated Cat and Cow: Placing your hands interlaced behind your head, do the Cat pose. Folding elbows forward, head slightly down and condense as you bring the elbows together in the front of the face with an exhale. Then open the folded arms, bringing the arms back along the shoulders with a slight arch back while inhaling. Repeat 5 sets

Side bends: Inhale and raise the left arm. Lean to the right, extending the arm overhead and to the right. Exhale and bring the arm back to the center. Repeat with the right arm over the head, bending to the left side and then back to center.

Seated twist: Find a comfortable seated posture facing forward. Turning to the right, bring the right arm behind you and hold the chair back. Continue rotating with the left hand twisting the torso and place the left hand on the outside of the right leg.

EARLY YOGA ACTIVITIES

Yoga for Toddlers age 18 months-3 years

Toddlers can imitate simple movements. Adults can assist using hands on, and verbal cues. Move slowly through the poses with a gentle voice and pace. Repeat several times or to tolerance. You may wish to offer a gentle touch and handling, to assist the child to get in and out of poses. Face the child or sit behind the child as you face a mirror.

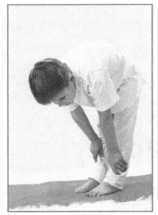
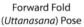

Forward Fold
(*Uttanasana*) Pose

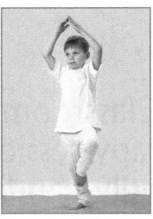

Tree Pose

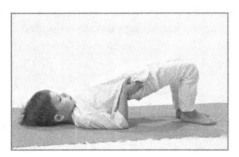

Bridge Pose

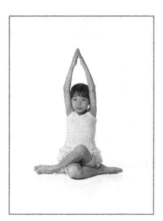

Cow Face

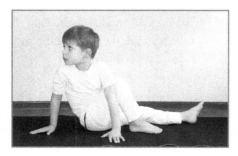

Seated Twist

Toddler's Standing Poses and Hands and Knee Poses

With toddlers, the therapist or caregiver needs to hold the child for support and may need to assist the child into the pose depending on age. Therapists can start working with a young child using yoga as early as infancy offering the opportunity to move through developmental patterns. Child's pose has the underpinnings of an early basic neuro-cellular pattern (a principle of Body Mind Centering) called a spinal pattern; the Downward Dog offers a chance for the therapist to assist the child to do upper body weight bearing and has the underpinnings of a push pattern. Facilitating Upward Dog develops the child's back and neck muscles. Other poses that can be facilitated are:

- Forward bend
- Tree
- Downward Facing Dog
- Upward Dog
- Three-legged Dog
- Bridge
- Cat
- Cow
- Child's pose
- Sponge pose

Seated Floor *Vinyasa* For Any Age

- Begin in Cobbler Pose.

- Crossing one leg over the other, stacking the knees pointed forward, place the calves and ankles on the sides of the thighs and directed back towards the hips and reach up with arms. Assume Cow Face Pose and inhale the arms up and exhale.

- Extending the legs forward straighten out, inhale the arms up and into a forward bend and exhale. Come back up to a seated pose. Inhale as you side-bend to right, weight-bear on right hand and left arm extends over head to right side. Repeat on opposite side.

- Place the left foot on the floor with knee bent and extend the right leg. Inhale as you twist to left and place left hand to floor behind left hip, then turn left and place right hand on the outside of the left knee on the floor or the leg. Exhale in the pose. Repeat on opposite side.

- End with Sponge Pose.

SENSORY AND YOGA CIRCLE TIME FOR PRESCHOOLERS

Sensory Yoga originated from serving populations of students with mixed skill levels in a group. Some students had sensory processing issues and needed extra cueing to be successful with a movement oriented circle time. As a preschool itinerant OT, I would offer to do 10 minutes of circle time. I would combine my experience of using sensory processing activities with yoga. I might add tasks that utilized the tactile system or touch and proprioception or information to the joints and vestibular or movement such as rocking. I coined the term "sensory yoga" when I added these qualities to an activity. Often teachers will welcome a break from the traditional circle time. Without going into a lot of detail with the teachers, I would explain how yoga could be helpful for self-regulation, reducing behaviors and movement skills for the class. I emphasized that breathing can help children's nervous systems switch from sympathetic to parasympathetic, explaining that this helps the kids become calmer. You can demonstrate this by doing several poses, deep breathing and a relaxation pose such as the Sponge.

GET STARTED USING SENSORY YOGA

- Suggest a "push–in" during preschool or school age circle.
- Explain that yoga is relaxing, includes breathing and reduces behavior issues.
- Note the preventive nature of body based focused activity.
- Promote how yoga can contribute to avoiding anxious behaviors.
- Use a visual image of a pose on a card, iPad, or notebook.
- Demonstrate the pose and ask the children to imitate you.
- Educate teachers with a yoga DVD of music and postures.
- Allow the children to become accustomed to the poses.
- Practice the sequence repeatedly in the same order.
- Embrace each child at their own pace and capability.
- Watch for tolerance and response to the calming ambiance.
- Choose a video, if needed that is calming and appropriate for your group.
- Beware of videos with fast images and distracting animation.
- Choose a temperately animated video.
- Utilize a sensory yoga group as preparation for seated work, before a rest time or as a break in the day between activities.
- Have fun with the results.
- Stay in the present moment, avoid judging the experience.

SENSORY YOGA GROUP FOR 3-5 YEAR OLDS

I have held many sensory yoga groups at preschools and school programs. The groups took place in an integrated classroom with typical and special needs children ages 3-5 years old. This 10-15 minute sequence was tolerated well. If you wish, you can add a longer relaxation in the last 2-3 minutes. Plan a 2-minute re-orientation and transition back to the circle time schedule. Allow for variance, depending on your group.

I always demonstrated the poses myself and had a picture to show the group. I would mix doing some sensory activities in with the poses. If the kids were lying on their stomachs, I might go around the circle and apply deep pressure with the large green ball on each child's back. Sometimes, one child demonstrated the pose along with me. It was evident that most children loved to do yoga poses that had an animal name. The children stay interested and want to move their bodies.

Walking around the circle, I held up a picture of each pose for the children to see. Keeping my voice quiet and gentle, I engaged the children by asking questions such as: "We are going to do a pose like a dog. Who has seen a dog stretch? Who has a dog at home? What is your dog's name?" This allowed me to stay engaged with the individual children and monitor who needed some extra attention. We would then do the pose of Downward Dog together. This also would meet some of the teacher's goals for the group for following directions, focusing and paying attention.

Doing circle time yoga in a group also revealed to the teacher and myself unidentified sensory processing issues or poor motor planning skills in the children. I would make a mental note of who couldn't follow the directions, wasn't able to distinguish between a command to lie down on their back or stomach, became overly excited or couldn't self-calm, I would mention my findings to the teachers and make suggestions for further evaluations if needed.

EQUIPMENT

- Medium size green therapy ball
- Small squishy koosh®
- Vibrating toy (optional)
- Pictures of the poses (on cards, iPad or a notebook)
- Bean bags for eye pillows, wash cloths or paper towel
- DVD if you prefer to not demonstrate

SCRIPT FOR PRESCHOOL SENSORY YOGA GROUP

"Today we will be doing some movement, breathing and imitating the shapes of animals with our bodies. Who wants to be an animal? At times we can make noise and other times we have to be very quiet. Before we start, I will be passing around the large green ball. When it is your turn, you can say your name and tap the ball as hard as you wish. After your turn, pass the ball to your friend and then sit very quietly. Show me you are ready by looking up here at me."

PROTOCOL FOR SENSORY YOGA

- Lights out or dimmed
- Lay mats or towels out in a circle
- Give children their own safe space
- Begin with a sensory warm up activity
- Breathe deeply (the equal breath teacher counts the beats out loud. Inhale 3, Exhale 3. Repeat 2-3 x)
- Practice poses
- Relax in Do-Nothing-Doll pose
- Sing

RATIONALE

- Proprioceptive activity "to tap the ball" helps some children settle down
- Introduce Mountain pose for line-up and for standing still
- Breathing activates the parasympathetic nervous system for calming
- Singing at the end of poses creates deep relaxation

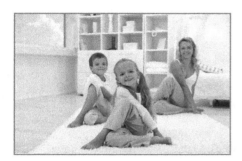

Pretzel Twist Pose

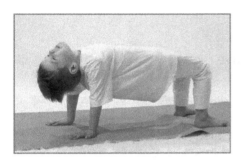

Table Pose

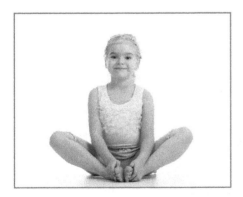

Butterfly (flutter knees) Pose

Preschool Poses

Start in a seated pose. Begin by having the children inhale and raise their arms. If you do a backbend always do a forward bend to follow and balance the body. Always do poses on both sides of the body. We always inhale as we arch, extend up and exhale as we flex, fold in and come down. These poses may be used for school-aged children through adolescents. If this sequence is too long for your client, you may shorten it.

- Pretzel twist
- Belly breathing or equal breath
- Cat and Cow
- Sphinx
- Downward Dog
- Upward Dog
- Tree
- Mountain
- Table
- Bridge
- Butterfly (flutter knees)
- Lion
- Child's pose
- Sponge pose
- Sing names of the students. Or design a song of calming, inspiring words such as: snowflakes falling silently, sun shines down on me.

Relaxation

- Sponge pose: Lie down on back in the Do-Nothing-Doll pose
- Lie on the back with arms relaxed and palms up, legs spread slightly
- Offer a blanket or sweater during sponge as children may become cold
- Increase the relaxation with bean bags or towels as eye pillows
- Allow the children to rest for several minutes after the poses

WHAT TO DO WITH CHALLENGING BEHAVIORS

Helper jobs: If a child Can't Follow the Poses

- Choose to allow the child to just be
- Give deep pressure or breathe by sitting back to back
- Have the child sit near you
- Create helper jobs for that child:
  - Lay out the mats
  - Roll the koosh ball under the students during Bridge, and Table
  - Hold up the pictures of the poses
  - Pass out the eye pads (bean bags or folded wash cloth, paper towel)
  - Identify if anyone is cold during Sponge pose/ Do-Nothing-Doll
  - Pass out blankets, towels or jackets during relaxation
  - Collect eye pads and blankets

IF THE CLASS GETS DISRUPTIVE

- Lower the lights
- Encourage everyone to lie down in Sponge pose
- Watch a yoga DVD and allow the children to watch or do the poses
- Accept what level of participation is possible
- Avoid demanding participation or punishing
- Pick very simple poses: Cat, Cow and Sponge pose
- Add sensory stimuli (Thera-Band® pull, vibration, straw-blowing tasks)
- Make the session shorter
- Permit low expectations
- Be happy with the results
- Practice non-judgment and acceptance with yourself and the students
- Praise the kids' involvement at what level they can do
- Read a story while the children lie in Sponge pose
- Patiently keep trying: Exposure to the calm ambiance is cumulative

TRANSITION BACK TO CIRCLE

- Instruct the children when Sponge is over to sit up slowly
- Script: "It is time to come back to the circle. We are coming to the end of our yoga session. Please sit up in a comfortable posture. We will sing . . ."
- Prepare children to end circle, with legs crossed
- Give the children the directions to "inhale."
- Give directions to: "Exhale while saying a word that is inspiring": courage, love, friendship etc. as a group in a singing fashion or the children can also say their name

Closing Variation 1

- Time is given for the transition, ending 5 minutes before the hour
- The children are asked to sit up quietly and listen for the next instructions
- The children sing out their names
- The instructor thanks the children for participating and putting mats away

Closing Variation 2

- The children place their hand together palms touching near their hearts
- Inhale and end with exhaling out the sound O as in "open."
- In a singing fashion sing out, "open our hearts "as they open their arms to the sides then squeeze the hand of the child near them. This can end the session or everyone together can take a bow together and say, "I bow to the light within you and me" or repeat "peace" three times as the closing ritual
- Children roll up mats and put away

Closing Variation 3

- Place the hands in a mudra touching thumb and first finger together
- Exhale the O sound
- Place hands on lap, the children bow to one another silently
- The children can repeat, "I bow to the light within you and me" silently or out loud and make eye contact with the group. Or, the teacher can say this for the group. Repeat the word "peace" 3 times to close.
- Children put the mats away.

ADAPTIVE YOGA FOR CLASSROOM AND CLINIC

Yoga can be used as a treatment modality and enhancer to meet many goals within a hospital, clinic or school setting. Adaptive yoga is a process by which we might alter a pose to the capability of the clients, with props or assistance. Whether we are trying to bend forward to pull socks up and choose to practice a seated version of forward bend, gain balance with Tree pose against a wall, or reduce anxiety with a hand mudra, yoga can be applied at any age to assist in learning daily living skills.

As an OT in the schools, I often suggested Mountain pose to teachers for children with sensory processing issues and with poor line-up skills. Teachers would often use it for the entire class.

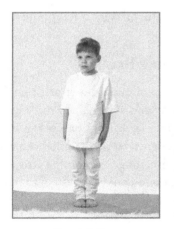

Mountain Pose

Line-Up Cues: Mountain Pose and Grounding Pole

- Ask the children to come to stand.
- Invoke the image of a mountain: still, strong, even and steady.
- Have the children stand in a natural pose, placing their arms at their sides, and feel their feet melt into the earth while standing straight.
- Imagine a grounding pole going from their feet down to the center of the earth holding them still and steady.

YOGA WITH PROFOUNDLY AUTISTIC AND PHYSICALLY HANDICAPPED INDIVIDUALS

In a school for autistic and profoundly handicapped children, a physical therapist was successful having a session using the following protocol:

- Secure a quiet space familiar to the student. (In this case, all the other students left the classroom for another activity, and the therapist worked at the circle time rug near where the student sat, so as not to disturb him.)
- Play quiet music (can use Pandora® Radio on the iPad®).
- Use a gentle soft voice and touch to communicate your presence.
- Use the same set routine of postures.
- Start with a seated pose on the floor, legs extended.
- The therapist sits facing the student with legs extended also.
- Therapist places her legs on the outside of the child's legs.
- Bending at the waist, the therapist pulls the student's arms gently creating a gentle rocking motion backward and forward.
- Facilitate the following sequence of poses for the child:
  ○ Happy Puppy (quadruped and rock hips laterally)
  ○ Cat and Cow
  ○ Child's pose
  ○ Tree pose with assistance
  ○ Happy baby
- Conclude with guided imagery meditation

USING THE BREATH TO HELP A STUDENT WITH CEREBRAL PALSY SELF-CALM

Patty is a bright teen who has cerebral palsy. She wears a scoliosis jacket, is tube fed, is non-verbal and uses an eye gaze-driven computer to communicate. One day, during my session, she was very uncomfortable and couldn't settle down. She was rejecting her fluid through the tube, and so we tried breathing together. She also liked it when I talked to her about anatomy, and put her hand on my bones and then placed her hand on her bones. We tapped the sternum and I asked her to focus on the front of the spine and the digestive tract. I took her hand and put it on my belly so she could feel me breathing. Then I put her hand on her own belly. Slowly she was able to lengthen her breath, relax, and accept the fluids.

APPLICATIONS OF THE ATTUNEMENT LIFESTYLE PROFILE: CULTIVATING BALANCE

The Attunement Lifestyle Profile (a self-processing tool) is an integrative or holistic group of questions to assist families or clients in assessing what might be needed to arrive at a healthy lifestyle in mind, body and spirit. The Profile can be helpful for any family and for those coping with the stress of raising a child who has trauma, sensory processing issues, autism or any special needs or just the typical stress of raising children. The profile is designed so that families can assess what strengths they have already, or have the potential for, and what areas need strengthening. The profile also offers in the questions some yogic and mindfulness principles that parents might not have realized could help them to reduce stress. Examples such as eating a meal together to encourage communication, taking time for silence and contemplation and everyone taking a break from electronics in the name of family time, can be vitally helpful for quality of life.

USING A SELF-PROCESSING TOOL WITH A SPECIAL NEEDS TEEN

Lucy is a 12-year-old girl who lost the use of both her legs. She uses a Hoyer lift for transitions, a motorized chair, and has good cognitive and verbal language skills. Lucy had spent the first 8 years of her life as neuro-typical and had an unfortunate situation that led to her disabled state. She could easily make her needs known and had conversations that a typical 12-year-old would have, although her articulation was slurred. At times it was difficult for others to understand what she wanted which was frustrating for her. She had one functional upper extremity, but the other affected arm didn't function as a consistent stabilizer. Lucy was more mature than her age due to her unusual transition to disability. She was observed helping other children in the house reach for things with her functional extremity and she clearly enjoyed that role.

During her occupational therapy intake for her group home, after covering the basic OT assessment areas, we discussed the profile with a staff member present. We looked together at the PowerPoint version of the Attunement Profile adapting it to the community and family milieu of the group home setting. The profile is available through a certification course and ebook: The Attunement Lifestyle Profile: Cultivating Balance taught by the author.

Lucy was able to see the pictures that accompany the questions. She looked carefully at each slide and took in the emotionality of the visuals. She was very interested in the visual slides and questions such as, "do you have family meetings?" "do you go on educational outings?" and, "do you have friends to laugh with?"

The house assistant supervisor and I gleaned many of Lucy's important feelings from the use of the profile. The conversation that ensued allowed us to problem solve in the moment. We identified possible options to enhance quality of life that the program already had in place but hadn't yet considered for Lucy. The profile shed light on Lucy's feelings at this time, and illuminated the subtleties of her lifestyle preferences. It was a true game changer and empowered Lucy and encouraged the staff to deliver quality services that were already available but not yet implemented for her.

TIPS AND TAKE AWAYS

- Maintain a sense of humor.
- Teach what you know.
- Keep the activity simple.
- Be compassionate with yourself and others.
- Strive to be even-keeled.
- Avoid punishing or getting angry during yoga.
- Go with the flow.
- Adapt to kids' tolerance.
- Remember less is more.
- Avoid rushing to get somewhere.
- Emphasize sensing, breathing, being, feeling, embodying.
- Create a safe space.
- Remember to breathe yourself.
- Focus on relaxation and acceptance.

When doing yoga with students, remember your own state of mind is the most important gift and the vehicle to a successful session or class for others. Being open, having fun and keeping things light is half the challenge. It is less about getting somewhere, and more about being where you are in each moment. If you need to calm yourself, take a few extra moments in the beginning with the client or class and together practice deep breathing. Get eye contact from the students, and be gentle in any handling techniques. One student I work with will only tolerate three repetitions of one moving warm-up pose. For him, that is an accomplishment, and I am happy with the response. When I practice contentment with the results no matter how small they are, the practice flows more easily.

CHAPTER 3

Guided Somatic Imagery in the Classroom and Clinic

GUIDED IMAGERY AND TRAUMA

Guided imagery is a tool I have used successfully with clients such as autistic young adults, trauma clients, and adults with panic attacks. I have also used guided imagery to help people with grieving, relaxation and caregiver burnout. Clients will share that they have felt totally rejuvenated or have experienced the reserves of universal consciousness.

A SELF-EXPLORATION ABOUT PHYSICAL PAIN USING GUIDED IMAGERY

Guided imagery has given me pertinent mind body information about myself through colors and images. Once I did an exploration about my hip which was feeling uncomfortable. During a self-guided imagery I saw an image arise that looked like broken scattered rocks. When I contemplated this, I realized I was experiencing enormous stress, because I had taken on too many projects and felt very scattered about my life. Only in a state of deep relaxation was I able to have that image surface for me to examine. Upon making some life changes, I was able to alleviate the stress and ultimately the physical discomfort.

SIMPLE IMAGERY CAN ASSIST US TO PROCESS FEELINGS.

I was walking the dog in the woods in my yard, expressing gratitude for the grace in my life and a passage that my daughter and I had moved through. I was also thinking about my book and a section I was re-writing about trauma. Nonchalantly, I threw my apple core into the woods. To my dismay my treasured bracelet of valuable stones flew off my hand at the same time. I witnessed and heard it land on the ground 10 feet away in the brush. It had been a beloved gift and I was shocked and disappointed and could barely process the loss. I attempted to find it but couldn't see the brown stones amongst the brown leaves and ground. But as I looked, my awareness shifted to go get a rake and as I did, I was also flooded with feelings about my house and a consideration I had about selling it. All of this increased awareness was coming from this incident. As I raked the ground and leaves searching I was able to accept I might not find the bracelet. It also felt okay that it had been released from me, as if I had arrived at a new passage in life and no longer needed it. The image of the rake also resonated with raking through what was important to me as if to gain clarity in preparation for my future transition. Although I felt sad about losing the bracelet and the feelings were still there, I saw and experienced the incident in a more transcendent way.

    In her book, *Invisible Heroes: Survivors of Trauma and How They Heal*, psychologist Belleruth Naparstek, explains how guided imagery has an impact on the brain: Trauma produces changes in the brain that impede a person's ability to think and talk about the event, but that actually accentuate their capacity for imaging and emotional-sensory experiencing around it. Imagery uses what's most accessible in the traumatized brain to help with the healing (p. 13).
When we do a guided somatization into the physical body systems we can help a traumatized client to connect the brain and body. We can then tune into what is accessible in the brain instead of disassociation. Just by merely exploring the physical body in this way and being fully present physically while tuning into feelings is a step towards healing.

Breathing with the Body Systems

The Body Mind Centering principle of layering through the body systems is utilized here.

- Give cues to breathe into the abdomen and organs
- Bring awareness to the three-part breath
- Notice how the breath moves through all three areas of the lower abdomen, lower lungs and chest as you inhale and exhale
- Notice the skin and the layers under the skin
- Notice the muscle and fascia
- Notice the bones and the fluids flowing within the body as you breathe gently
- Notice all the cells that make up the body
- While lying supine, notice your spine and the relationship of your head and tail or the sacrum down to the coccyx bone
- Notice the pelvic halves on each side
- Place your hands on your hips and feel the large bones
- Feel the ribcage and notice it is the outer container for the lungs and organs

SOMATIC EXERCISES FOR TRAUMA

When working with a client with trauma, the activities below may be explored to prepare the client for a somatic oriented experience when combined with deep breathing.

Find these activities in the book to explore this work further:

- Guided imagery
- Slow seated chair *Vinyasa*
- *Savasana* (Sponge pose)
- Restorative poses (legs on wall)
- Hip Rotation Clock Face

Guided imagery is a right brain technique that engages the emotions, senses and imagination. Some people use the terms guided visualization and guided imagery interchangeably. The main point is that the exercise is *guided*. This means another person is speaking and suggesting images that are meant to engage all of the participant's senses: typically feeling, hearing, seeing, smelling and sometimes taste. Another element is that there is a beginning, middle and end in the imagery. Guided imagery has been proven to have health benefits and create relaxation. In this next section, I will be describing a guided imagery sequence and moving warm-ups that I used in a multi-handicapped classroom. The activities below can be used for any client's goal to achieve relaxation, a sense of safety, connection to self and to provide deep rest. Although I refer to children in the activity it applies to any age group. Below I describe using guided imagery with autistic young adults at a school yoga session.

This simple sequence with breathing and guided imagery had a huge impact. We used moving warm-ups of raising and lowering contralateral arms and legs movements in supine. Instructions were given to the group to inhale and exhale which helped the group to relax and cease making noises and rocking.

Here is an activity that was successfully used for this population in a classroom on Halloween after all the festivities in a class at a school. In the morning, all the kids and staff had dressed in costume, and each class had prepared a unique activity. We went around putting hands into mushy goo, throwing apples, playing smart board games and getting tattoos. There was a lot of sensory overload, screaming and stimulation. Everyone's energy plummeted after this, and the day slowed to a snail's pace. When it was time for yoga, we realized the DVD wouldn't be available. I offered to teach the yoga class to all the students and the staff. Everyone was so exhausted. I decided to do relaxation instead of poses. I started my guided imagery exercise, which evolved into an embodied meditation. The kids really embraced the activity and became completely still. Within 15 minutes of the guided imagery, everyone had relaxed on his or her mat in supine. The result was that we couldn't hear a peep, or any movement, just stillness in the room.

Depending on the group and their movement ability, I might start with moving warm-ups to relax the physical body and prepare for the imagery exercise.

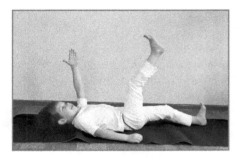

Moving Warm–Ups

Moving Warm–Ups

The Embodyoga principle of moving warm-ups is utilized here.

1. Extend both arms overhead while in supine with an inhale.

2. Exhale as you return the arms to the sides of the body.

3. Repeat moving the arms several times with an inhale and exhale.

4. Raise the arms and legs the right arm and right leg, left arm, left leg.

5. Incorporate connecting the body from the fingertips to the toes.

6. Imagine a ray of light passing from fingertips down to the toes and through the spine. Let the ray of light extend out of all the limbs.

7. The blue light starts at the right fingers and travels all the way to the left toes. Stretch as you are imagining the light.

8. Repeat this with the other side.

Guided Imagery: The Floating Raft

- Invite the children to imagine they are floating on a raft.
- Describe the color of the water, the gentle rocking movements, the sun on the face, the smells and the wind.
- Use evocative and sensory rich language, words such as yielding, floating, and melting into the earth.
- Suggest that they let the back of the body yield into the floor as they lie on their mat. Yielding is like a melting sensation; letting the weight of their body go.
- Suggest they imagine the wind blowing against them as they travel in the raft.
- Ask them to explore the beautiful scenery, such as green covered mountains and blue sky, and enjoy the gentle rocking of the raft as they float.
- Suggest that the raft returns to the edge of the land and it is time to get out and start walking home.

Guided Imagery: The Steps

This is not an exact script, but a sequence with guidelines, and may work as a script for you. Make the words your own when instructing a group, but first read through to the end before using it.

- Imagine walking through a field.

- Suggest sensing all the flowers, colors, smells, the sun and feeling the grass.

- See a staircase that goes up.

- We are walking up 20 steps. Take an inhale on a step and an exhale on the next step until the 20 steps are finished.

- Describe the scene with sounds and colors. For example, say: "At the top of the steps, listen to the waterfall. See lush green-covered mountains, trees with new green leaves of spring, and a flowing river below."

- Walk slowly down the concrete steps closer to the river and listen to the waterfall.

- Walk down 20 steps with an inhale and exhale on each step.

- Describe the scene at the bottom of the steps, the trees, landscape, smells, and colors. For example: "At the bottom of the steps the clear river flows and on it, a boat passes by. Palm trees, giant ferns and cows graze in the high grass in the distance. Sit on a bench to rest."

Guided Imagery: Seeing an Old Friend

In this guided meditation we meet an old friend. It may be used with adults, adolescents and for children. It offers the experience of reconnecting to relationships that may have been interrupted due to trauma. We might feel the loss of a loved one due to relocation, illness, loss of a friendship or family member, divorce, violence, and death. The opportunity to have a positive experience with a loved one in a guided imagery is very soothing and can bring a joyful satisfaction to the client.

- Imagine seeing an old friend sitting on a bench along the river.

- Meet and greet your old friend.

- Reach for your friend's hand.

- Join the friend at the bench and sit together.

- Remind the group how good it feels to see an old friend.

- Drop into the heart as you sit with your friend. Feel the feelings that come up.

- Look lovingly into your friend's eyes and face.

- Ask a question or share your feelings with your friend.

- Pause for a moment for your friend's answer to reveal itself

- Savor the quiet moment with your friend.

- It is now time to say goodbye to your friend and start the journey home.

- Get up from the bench, hug your friend goodbye, and walk away contentedly.

- Emphasize we are just leaving "for now."

- Remind everyone that we can come back to visit this place again.

The Journey Home

When it is time to transition back to the classroom, here are some tips for ending the guided imagery:

- Introduce an ending to the guided meditation: "Walk back to the field, find the raft, float back and get out."

- Invite everyone to slowly open their eyes and come back to the room.

- Allow time for transition after such a deep meditative state. Plan for the meditation directions to close 5 minutes before the end of the session to allow for ample transition time, so that people don't have to pop up, but can linger and enjoy the fruits of this restful experience.

- Some participants may be sleeping and need gentle cues to wake up or you might want to let them rest and have planned ahead for that response.

NOTES TO REMEMBER:

- Do yoga at the same time every week or every day.

- Roll out the mats and ask for the students to participate.

- Remove children from the wheelchairs to the mat.

- Give support with a prop to position the child in a comfortable position.

- Instruct staff to sit next to the students.

- Invite staff to use a soothing touch that is therapeutic and appropriate to the setting you are in to calm the children if they wish.

- Offer a therapeutic touch on a student's hand, arm, leg, back or stomach.

- Encourage staff and students to lie down on the mats.

- Invite everyone to "find a place in the body to be comfortable."

- It is preferable to do a set of moving warm-ups in the beginning only and not after you have started the guided imagery as it can counter the meditation.

- Speak in a gentle quiet voice.

- Invite all the participants to inhale to a count of 4 and exhale for a count of 4.

- Encourage students to lie supine, side lie or sit.

- Encourage staff to participate 100 % for the full yoga and guided imagery.

TIPS AND TAKE AWAYS

Trauma Sensitive Yoga Precautions

The somatic guided imagery exercises described in this chapter may be used for any age or classroom and adapted to special populations or trauma. **In being sensitive to trauma, it is important to not hold any restorative pose for an extended time with a trauma client**. This can cause discomfort to a trauma client. If you use the pose **only hold it for a minute or two**.

This can be adjusted as you check for feedback with your clients. An extended restorative pose for 15-20 minutes that is used in yoga restorative class is not appropriate in this context for a trauma client as it might tend to bring up too many feelings that are overwhelming for the client and they are left for too long unattended in a stationary pose.

I have used it with adults in my workshops and it has brought a deeply satisfying experience of rest and rejuvenation. These exercises have also been used successfully in a multi-handicapped, autistic, non-verbal young adult classroom ages 14-21, with good receptive language skills. For children who don't have good receptive language skills, just use very simple images.

Encoding tissue memories with timing and staff participation

Keeping a scheduled time for yoga is beneficial. This helps the students to know what to expect and for the body to encode the memories on the somatic and cellular levels from week to week. The body will store the memory of the relaxation as it clears out more and more tension. The experience can have a cumulative impact as the child begins to learn to breathe from the belly, to follow the cues of the group leader, and to allow and trust the relaxation to occur.

In a special needs classroom, when staff participated in the relaxation, I found that the children had a deeper relaxation experience.

- Invite the staff to close their eyes and participate if permitted.
- If you are in a special needs setting and if it's appropriate, and meets the students' needs, I suggest encouraging the staff to lie down, and to calmly place one hand on the student in a therapeutically acceptable way to give tactile input.
- Follow all safety regulations and school protocol as needed.
- As you lead the group in the guided imagery, dim the lights and use a soft voice.
- Low gentle music can be played in the background.

I found this to be a successful template for young adult special needs students with good receptive language, even if they were non-verbal. They were able to follow the breathing directions and became very quiet and relaxed.

- When we offer a guided imagery, it may be short or long depending on the participants' tolerance.
- It can be simple such as swimming with Nemo® and seeing fish and sea life.
- Engage the mind with as many images such as visual, embodied cues, temperature, nature, auditory, gustatory and olfactory images.
- This allows us to have an emotional and somatic response.

Meet the relaxation state of the group

Guided imagery offers so many rich opportunities to help students relax into meditation and reconnect to their somatic self. Whether it is simple or more complex, imagery can root and route us through the senses back to an awareness of our source. There might be a tendency to underestimate the impact of a guided imagery session. As you practice instructing guided imagery, you will gain confidence as you see participants relax, slow their breathing and the room become still. **Be aware of the energy in the room changing from the guided meditation**. I have sensed a palpable stillness that signals to me that the participants are engaged and have shifted into a relaxation state. I then check in with my own breathing and meet the relaxation state of the group's experience. Then, I can be deeply sensitive to the experience that the group is having and lead what is needed to end the session.

CHAPTER 4

Nature and Somatic Learning

RECONNECTING CHILDREN TO NATURE

I can remember as a child having a 10-minute walk from the house to my elementary school building. Getting to school involved traveling on a blacktopped path, fenced in on both sides, through a wooded area that had defied development. We entered from a cul-de-sac, and the entrance of the path had houses with bright colors and we smelled flowers. The path descended down through undeveloped wooded land, sloped slightly down to the bottom then flattened out. It ascended a hill to come out into the schoolyard. I probably had more experiences on that path, than I can remember from my grammar school classes.

We had experiences of how our bodies felt, which years later I recognized as somatic experiences. We would stop for a minute where the path flattened out to look into the woods and to watch nature. We listened to the birds, made snowballs and threw them. We stomped in the puddles, slid down the icy hill, before facing the reality of the schoolyard. We stopped to gossip, to harmlessly tease and grab a friend's hat. Or chase a friend up the hill to the schoolyard.

On an icy morning, the boys would deliberately fall down on the hill and push each other. The children played physically: body-slammed, bounced, fell, and arrived at school with their snow suits caked in snow. We had to step carefully to avoid the mud in the spring. We would pause in the fall to be astonished by a brilliantly colored fallen red leaf on the path, but we couldn't dawdle too much and arrive late.

Many sensory, cognitive learning and proprioceptive inputs filled the early morning walk to school. We climbed the hill with our book bags, bouncing into the fence at times attempting to climb it. The fence's construction had some give in it, and it moved if your body slammed it. We elbowed one another up the path as more kids came to walk with us to avoid being left behind the group. We grasped and pulled on the fence down the hill to not slide or fall. We stepped carefully to avoid puddles, (or to make sure you landed in one). We strategized our upward climb to arrive without falling.

QUIETING THE MIND THROUGH NATURE

Our walk provided a somatically rich morning, socially, cognitively, and in movement. Being in nature quieted our minds naturally before the school day started. We had ample opportunities to work out our stress physically. We arrived at school feeling our bodies. There was the inner warmth of arms and leg muscles that had exercised up the hill. The walk provided our senses with treasured experiences. We had seen real colors in nature, smelled the woods, and possibly tasted snowflakes.

VALUE TIME IN NATURE AS SKILL BUILDING FOR THE BRAIN

My own childhood experiences inspired me to provide ample outside activities for my family. As a therapist, I would use outside play as much as possible, inviting families to meet me at the playground modeling to parents this type of play. Often, a parent would think their child was incapable of navigating the swings or slide, only to discover an enthusiastic and capable child. Often, it was the parent who was holding back out of a sense of protectiveness. Once the parent could see how able the child was, they were more eager and open to more vigorous outside play.

These lovely nature and social experiences for children are priceless. But for many, they may not be available. The concern over violence has changed the way we live, and we are not as carefree as we once were. I wouldn't let my grammar school child walk unattended through a wooded area nowadays. However, we can certainly try to duplicate these outside nature experiences. Many parents do carefully plan outside time. Unfortunately, for many children, there is a lack of outside experiences. Yet, it is so important to have these sensory nature experiences, such as hiking, sledding, tubing and nature events, or a walk to school.

USE NATURE INSTEAD OF SCREENS TO REDUCE STRESS AND NURTURE THE BRAIN

But for many children, it is more common to go from watching a screen to the bus, to watch another screen possibly, to the class where there are also computers and then back home to a screen. It has now been noted that children are spending up to seven hours a day on screens, according to a new Kaiser Foundation study. The children in that study also appear to have lower grades in school.

I can remember an interaction with a well-meaning parent. She wanted to know if I thought she should allow her five-year-old to play outside immediately upon returning from school. The mother was concerned the child should finish her homework first. I explained the positive sensory impact of being outside in nature. After a stressful day at school, outside play for a five-year-old is healing for the brain. Children perform better with a physical break after school.

For many children, nature experiences aren't part of the fabric of living. For those children fortunate enough to spend time outside, parents often over schedule activities. The result is that children have less and less down time or unstructured play. There isn't enough of an outlet for our children's stress in everyday living. When outside time, gym, recess or afterschool activities, are eliminated we are left with fewer options to neutralize the effects of all those screens.

My concern for children's dwindling nature opportunities led me to explore how yoga and mindfulness might help reverse this. We can bring back nature and somatic experiences instead of spinning off-course with the stress of living daily. The activities in this book can be done at home, in classrooms and clinics.

Open-eyed Meditation in Nature: Allowing Joy to Emerge

- When your child or teen is having a difficult time, it can be very helpful to get out in nature and clear the mind with a walk. Staying in the present moment, while being in nature, is a healing activity for the mind and body. It gives young people time to take a break from electronic devices, get oxygen to the brain, and move the physical body. Optimal places are: a park, a playground, forest, mountain, lake, the ocean, a college campus or a trail. If you can't access nature then this can also be done on a city street. Biking is also an option. If there is no access to nature just get out and walk as you can. Trust your own intuition and what you feel attracted to on your walk. Stop to notice trees, sounds, water, flowers, birds or dogs. Allow the mind that is over-thinking or is in disharmony to open to the space around you.

- Make a point not to discuss problems with your child during this time. Allow the child to initiate talking. This may or may not happen and either way it's ok. The key point is to stay in the present moment without any goals.

- Allow your child the safe space to feel comfortable being in his or her body while doing this active exercise.

- Creating an activity that a child and an adult can do together without words (resonating in tune with one another silently) is very supportive for the child or teen. By letting go of the need to talk, we get nourishment from nature and silence. Use this opportunity to allow the mind, body, and the individual cells to regain balance and nourishment from nature.

- Tune into the body as you walk, noticing how your feet hit the ground, how your body is feeling.

Recommendations:

- After significant exercise, stop and rest in the silence that is created.
- Make an effort to respect and allow for the silence.
- If your child wants to be quiet, avoid initiating nervous chatter.

- Use the mindfulness practices. Your teen will notice the state of calm you are experiencing, as you practice acceptance, and non-judgment.

- If your child speaks, just listen and be appropriate in response.

- Hold the stillness of the moment. This is meditation in action. The mind becomes quiet on its own from physical exercise and from shifting the focus from thinking to the breath.

TIPS AND TAKE AWAYS

- While walking, use the time to watch your breath as you inhale and exhale. A simple way to do this is to focus your attention on the air as it comes in and out of your nose. When you experience resistance to doing this, just notice your resistance and gently bring the focus back to the breath.

- It isn't necessary to try to talk. Be in nature and allow the outside physical exercise to naturally calm the child's nervous system. Also, don't try to instruct your teenager in this method. Just being in nature together is enough. If the adult concentrates on their breathing, this will also support the teen energetically.

Being in nature for fun, to quiet my mind and get in touch with my feelings is a common way for me to spend time living in a small town in the mountains. When she was younger, I would often take my moody child walking in the woods. As a parent, I frequently made the mistake of asking questions at the wrong time when it would have been better to remain silent. The questioning would shut the conversation down. When I simply repeat a mantra, remained contented, relaxed, and focused on my breathing, my child would start to talk to me. Practicing "breathing into stillness", and time in nature allowed us to have better communication. (See Chapter 5)

CHAPTER 5

Pranayama Fills the Gap

Children need other skills beyond reading, writing, and math to make it in today's world. Without discarding the critical basics for education, we now need to include being intuitive, thinking out of the box and being compassionate with one another. We need to help children to cope with stress. Using mindfulness and a somatic approach, we can become more receptive and compassionate to ourselves and others.

Yoga provides a deeply needed "embodied" connection through the mind, body, senses and breath that can help improve academic skills and reduce stress. I understand this as needing to have a sixth sense. This can occur when we stay embodied or present, even-keeled, focused and intuitive. This helps us to embrace others and ourselves with compassion and understanding. We start this embodied exploration with experiencing *Pranayama*.

Pranayama means yogic breathing exercises that allow the universal life force or "*prana*" to flow freely. So by practicing deep breathing we can remove the stress of daily living and establish the flow of the breath to support us.

BREATHING INTO STILLNESS

As a teacher, the most important element in creating a healing space for yourself and others is to become established and grounded in the breath. Focus your attention on the air coming in and out of your nose while allowing your other thoughts to gently pass by. This simple but profound task will regulate you. If you are in a classroom, invite others to do this breathing. As the adults in the room focus on breathing, it creates a positive atmosphere for students in the room. This stillness seeps into the consciousness of the space around you. It makes a cushion for everyone in the room like a cocoon of positive energy. Instead of thinking "I am breathing for myself," breathe for everyone. Breathe your way into stillness. This very simple and practical technique can be used at work, school or home. Without anyone noticing what you are doing, you are supporting and maintaining harmony for yourself and those around you.

Breathing Into Stillness

- Hold your finger under your nose.
- Closing your mouth begin to inhale and exhale normally.
- Focus all your attention on the air coming in and out of your nose.
- As your mind drifts, or feels resistant, gently guide it back to the breath.
- Let the thoughts pass in the mind and refocus on the breath.
- Repeat 10-20 sets of inhale and exhale.
- Remove the finger and let yourself try breathing without the tactile cue.

Understanding Breathing

Leslie Kaminoff and Amy Matthews in their book, *Yoga Anatomy* share the analogy of a water balloon and an accordion to explain breathing.

- Use a water balloon that is filled only partially.
- Let the kids press and shape the water from the bottom of the balloon to the middle and then the top.
- Demonstrate how the breath moves through the belly or abdominal cavity.
- Show how the water moves yet stays within the border of the balloon.
- Demonstrate how the thoracic cavity, which can be compared to an accordion or a slinky toy, bellows in and out. Dividing the abdominal and thoracic cavities is the diaphragm, which is like a parachute shape.
- Notice how breathing is like an accordion sitting on top of a water balloon.
- Visualize the lungs, and belly chambers using these images.
- Alternately, you can use PlayDoh®, drawing or rolling paper wads into a sock and pushing the wads up or down to demonstrate the movement of the breath.
- Show how the air moves into various chambers.

The Three-Part Breath (See the Belly Elevator)

- Invite the children to lie down on their backs. (This can also be done seated).
- Ask them to place one hand on their belly and one on the chest.
- Notice how the stomach extends out with the inhale, and in with the exhale.
- Place a cotton ball, Koosh ball, tissue or a toy animal on the child's belly.
- Watch the object move up on an inhale and down with an exhale.
- Feel the air moving into the lower, middle and upper lobes.
- Put your hands on the ribs to feel the expansion and contraction.
- Have the child feel for the clavicle (collar bone).
- Notice how the clavicle moves up subtly on the last top lung chambers.
- Invite the children to comment about how they feel.

Belly Down Breathing

- Children can try belly down breathing while lying prone on their stomachs.
- Place the hands stacked under the forehead to rest the head as you practice.
- Feel how the air moves differently in the belly as you inhale and exhale.
- Ask the children what they feel.

Ujjayi Breath-Ocean Sounding Breath

Ujjayi breath is called ocean-sounding breath because we make a hissing sound or a throaty "ha" in the throat that sounds like the ocean on the exhale. To learn this breath we teach it with the mouth open. When we practice *Ujjayi*, we close the mouth, which makes the sound appear softer.

- Open the mouth and breathe out a throaty ha/hiss sound from the back of the throat that sounds similar to a gargle or a soft motor and sounds like the ocean. (It reminds me of the sound of holding a conch shell to your ear)
- After practicing several times, try it with the mouth closed.
- Practice the *Ujjayi* breath with the mouth closed until you feel comfortable with it.

Humming Bee Vibration Breath

The Humming Bee breath is a fun breath for any age child to learn, because they can make a sound, it has vibration and it feels like a sensory activity. The instructor can tell the story of the origin of the name of Humming Bee breath. In India, children were told a story that the Humming Bee breath occurred when a bee was humming inside your mouth. Invite the children to watch you do the Humming Bee breath demo first so they have a visual picture of it.

Therapist Demo of Humming Bee Breath

- Start to hum with your mouth closed.
- Place your fingers on your ears and close off the sound.
- Cover the eyes and close off the vision.

Instructions For Students' Practice of Humming Bee Breath

- Instruct the children to make a humming sound in their throats.
- Once they can hear the hum, instruct them to close their eyes.
- Placing fingers gently in their ears, ask them to close off the ears
- Gently close off the outside sounds. Gently experiment to find the right closure of the ear.
- Try out different tones of humming to see which one they like.
- Remember: Give instructions before the eyes and ears close.
- Try rounds of this fun sensory breath with various low and high tones.
- Invite the children to share their experiences.

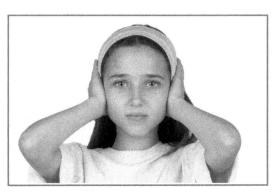

Humming Bee Breath Pose

Breathing with Embodied Cueing

- Give cues to breathe into the abdomen and organs.
- Bring awareness to the three-part breath.
- Notice how the breath moves through all three areas of lower abdomen, lower lungs and chest as you inhale and exhale
- Notice the skin and the layers under the skin.
- Notice the muscle and fascia.
- Notice the bones and the fluids flowing, the heart within the body.
- While lying supine notice your spine and the relationship of your head and tail or the sacrum down to the coccyx bone.
- Notice the pelvic halves on each side.
- Place your hands on your hips and feel the large bones.
- Feel the rib cage and notice it is the outer container for the lungs and organs.

CHAPTER 6

Embodied Learning

SENSORY YOGA FEELING WHEEL

My friend and I were talking while on our daily walk. We were talking about, the Wheel of Awareness, a concept created by Dr. Dan Siegel. She was sharing about her anxiety, hormone imbalances and physiological discomfort. I shared about how feelings are nuanced during the day and how to watch for the nuances rather than wait for the highs and lows. I wanted to give her some options rather than hovering around the same group of uncomfortable feelings of overwhelm. After our walk, we sat in the car with a scrap paper and an orange fine tipped marker and made the "Feelings Circle." In the middle, I put her name. Along the rim of the outer larger circle, we drew smaller circles. I asked my friend to give me words or feelings that made her happy and brought joy to her heart. She named cooking, puttering, her children, husband, gardening, and moving furniture. I wrote them down and placed the words in the smaller circles. I showed her how she can "shift the wheel" of her mind from the section that describes her anxiety to the more uplifting thoughts and activities.

PROPRIOCEPTIVE TASKS CALM THE NERVOUS SYSTEM

My friend shared that she loves moving furniture around the house. I explained that moving furniture is a "proprioceptive activity" because it brings feedback through the muscles and joints, which then is calming for the nervous system. Back home, I puttered around, embodying my senses as I unpacked my groceries. I smelled the daffodils, the fresh lemon, and enjoyed the bright red color and smell of the tomatoes. I felt calmer from the proprioceptive walking, carrying groceries and the "puttering" which became a moving meditation. This experience led me to add more somatic, yoga and sensory components while creating the Sensory, Yoga, and Feeling Wheel. The body-based activities can also be used in the classroom to help children become more grounded and act as an antidote to anxiety, fear and discouragement.

HOW TO USE THE SENSORY YOGA FEELING WHEEL

In the example below, the top circle demonstrates the child's anxiety or pre-occupying thought and feeling. This child is scared of a test. In the circles that go around clockwise are thoughts that are positive, uplifting and safe images to counter the negative fear. In all the circles including the top, are yoga and sensory activities to help shift the negative feelings with a body-based repair. All the activities use breathing, yoga and movement to shift the child's nervous system from the sympathetic to the parasympathetic. All the activities are somatic, layering the sensory experiences into the body on a cellular level as they combine with the breathing.

- You may wish to refer to the section on Witnessing the Mind (Chapter 9).
- Incorporate yoga and sensory components in all circles.
- Record the child's stressful event, fear or anxiety in the top circle.
- Place in each circle one or two yoga poses, breathing, sensory, or somatic activities
- Elicit from the child three or more positive thought constructs to ground him in safe, enjoyable and pleasant memories or activities.

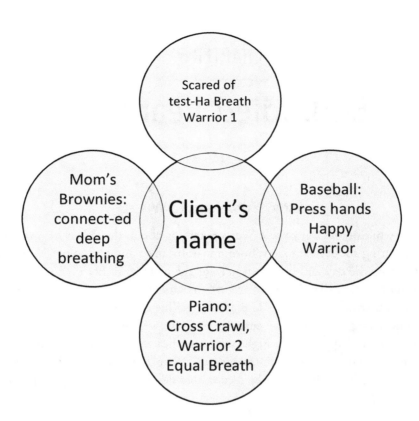

- Write one positive thought concept in each of the other circles.
- Engage body, mind, and spirit when choosing treatment modalities.
- Place the child's name in the center of the circle.
- Utilize sensory and somatic activities in the other three circles.
- Moving clockwise, engage in the yoga poses, crossing midline, and proprioceptive activities that accompany the positive as seen in the example.
- The last circle has breath, taste and smell (to foster connection to the limbic brain)
- A restorative pose or Do-Nothing-Doll can be added to aid in the relaxation.

HOW TO DO THE SAMPLE ACTIVITIES IN THE SENSORY YOGA FEELING WHEEL

The Ha Breath
- Do the Ha breath standing or seated.
- Place one leg forward about hip width apart into a comfortable lunge position, front foot facing forward and back foot at 45-degree angle.
- Gently bend knees slightly.
- Inhale the arms up fully, extending the arms up alongside the ears.
- Making the hands into fists, simultaneously while exhaling, pull the arms down, elbows to sides and say "Ha" loudly while bending the knees comfortably.

Same-Side Brain and Hand

The Body Mind Centering principle of body halves and brain registration is demonstrated in this activity. Bonnie Bainbridge Cohen, its founder, believes movement and the body inform the brain. While working on a post-stroke patient, Bonnie found that working with the non-affected leg and accessing the same-side brain, gave the patient movement in the affected side. This activity can be facilitated or done by the student independently.

- Share a picture of an outline of the lungs' shape.

- Starting with the right side, invite the child to push the right palm of hand together against the therapist's hand on the right side loading the input to one side only. The child can also place her right hand briefly on her own right shoulder. Then remove the hand from the shoulder.

- The therapist gives the client tactile input at the lung of the right side, or the client imagines the lungs and breathes into the lung giving him input.

- Breathe with the awareness of the three lobes.

- Become aware of the right brain half only, and try to access it (same side).

- Practice the activity of moving just the right arm, without crossing midline and stay within the right side of the body half only. Include the right lung as you move, feeling the difference of using the organs in movement.

- Cross midline with the right arm as you access the right side of the brain noticing the difference when you cross midline.

- Make a distinction between one body half first before trying it on the other side. Move slowly, then more dramatically, to get a sense of the body half.

- Repeat on the left side.

- Notice how it feels to access the same side brain half with same side movement. Notice how it feels to access the right side brain and cross midline to the left side movement.

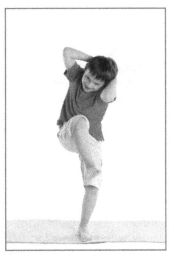

Cross Crawl Pose

Cross Crawl

- After you have given input with the palms pressing and accessing same side arm, lung and brain half, then attempt this step.

- Imagine the opposite brain side giving strength to the opposite body side.

- Lifting the left knee, bring right hand to touch it, repeat on opposite side, crossing midline.

- Variations include: touch opposite elbow to knee or lifting the bent leg behind the body, and touching the foot with opposite hand.

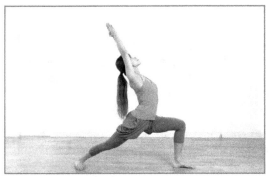

Warrior 1 Pose

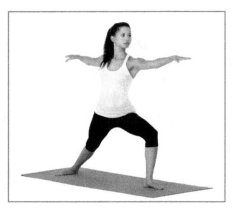

Warrior 2 Pose

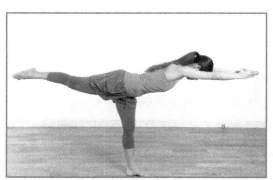

Warrior 3 Pose

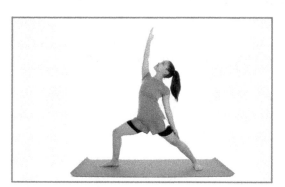

Happy Warrior Pose

Warrior Series

Yoga poses Warrior series (*Virabhadrasana*) 1,2,3 and Happy Warrior are all possible poses.

Warrior 1

Stand with feet and body facing forward. Extend your arms overhead and bend the right front knee as you step backwards with left leg. The front leg deepens with a bend into a lunge position. Maintain the foot and knee in alignment over one another. Extend the arms straight upward. Repeat on the other side.

Warrior 2

Take a wide stance facing the long side of your mat. Turn the front foot to 90° and the back leg to 30-45°. Your feet can be on the mat aligned under your hands. Let your sitz bones sink down and yield the feet into the floor. The back hip turns inward to the navel, and the front hip turns and spirals outward. The line between the feet and up to the sitz bones would make a perpendicular line. Plant the feet firmly as you sink down into the sit bones to ground you solidly. Extend the arms strongly over the feet and yield and bend the front leg sinking into a bent knee pose. The front knee is over the front foot. Repeat on the other side.

Warrior 3

Stand in *Tadasana* or Mountain pose. Inhale, lifting one leg and while exhaling, bend forward and balance on the one standing leg as you extend the opposite leg behind you in the air. Holding your arms extended in front, join the hands, palms facing one another to a full arm extension. Repeat on the other side.

Happy Warrior

Assume the Warrior 2 Pose. Inhale, lifting your front arm towards the sky, move it backwards, with the palm facing you. Take a slight backbend as you exhale and follow your palm with your eyes. Hold the posture. Smile for the Happy Warrior. Repeat on the other side.

Connect-ed

- Cross the left leg over the right at ankles. (You may wish to cross right).
- Place your hands, palms facing and touching upward, at chest level.
- Bring your left wrist over the right wrist closer to your chest.
- Turn the palms to face each other and interlace the fingers.
- Touch your tongue to the roof of your mouth and breathe deeply for one minute.
- Releasing the hands and tongue, return to palms-up position.

The Equal Breath

The equal breath involves silently counting and measuring the length of the inhale and exhale. It is an easy technique for any age. In this image the child is sitting in the Lotus pose.

- Sit in a comfortable position or lie in supine.
- Count to four counts and monitor the length of time as you inhale.
- Count as you exhale for four counts.
- Repeat increasing the inhale and exhale to five counts.
- Continue to increase breath up to six counts. (eight for adults with large lung capacity).

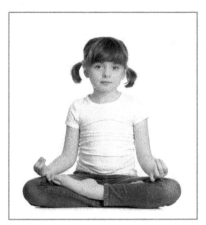

Equal Breath Pose

Therapeutic Interventions for Equal Breath

- Auditory cues:

  Use clapping hands, tambourine, tapping with pencil or drumsticks.

- Tactile cues:

  Add input as the therapist squeezes the client's hand for each count.

- Verbal

  Count to four with your voice or instruct to count silently.

- Visual cue

  Imagine a color as you inhale and exhale.

- Imagery cues

  Imagine smelling a flower, chocolate or a favorite scent.

- Olfactory cue

  If needed, you may wish to have the child smell something in order to participate. Use discretion in choosing a pleasant mild scent that will not distract or be overly stimulating. Maintain that the intention of the activity is to experience an inhale for a determined count of inhale and exhale.

THERAPIST TIPS FOR SENSORY YOGA FEELING WHEEL

1. Encourage the client to be spontaneous when making up the sensory yoga feeling wheel and the positive thoughts. The therapist might ask, "what are some things that you like to do?"

2. Help students to think of activities that involve a somatic experience. For an example, the therapist can say, "I like how my body feels when I sing, run or bowl." Then ask the child "What do you enjoy doing that makes your body feel good? Aim for responses that are more about "being and doing" than related to passively watching screens.

3. Add in favorite sensory modalities, deep pressure, vibration, movement.

Somatic Exercises for Trauma

When working with clients with trauma, the hand mudras and *Pranayama* exercises are very helpful. You may like to try with clients Activity: Breathe with Embodied Cueing. Give cues to breathe into the abdomen and organs. Suggested activities for a one-on-one session are found throughout the book.

- Guided imagery (See Chapter 3).
- Slow seated chair *Vinyasa*.
- Hand mudra: Tulip.
- *Savasana* (Sponge pose).
- 1-2 minute holding of Restorative poses only. Long holds are not indicated for a trauma client. (Legs on Wall).

Tick-Tock How Slow is your Clock. (Explore the Pelvic Floor)

In this exercise we explore how the body feels moving slowly and shifting weight through the pelvic bones. This is a powerful activity and can bring up feelings especially if you are moving slowly. It can also help with joint discomfort as it unlocks emotional holding. Working slowly can open us emotionally and is grounding. Exploring the pelvic floor and diaphragm is relaxing and helps us to let go of muscular tension. On a chair, pretend you are sitting on a clock. Recognize where the 12, 6, 3, 9 would be located.

- Put hands on hips, and feel the large bones of the two pelvic halves.
- Notice the "sitz bones" or ischial tuberosity, the bony prominence at the bottom of the hipbone, which you are sitting on.
- Gently rock between 3 and 9 o'clock to feel where the sitz bones are located.
- Gently move in the diagonal from 1 to 7 and 11 to 5.
- Gently move slowly around the entire clock, starting at 12 clockwise.
- Use the equal breath to slow down the breathing and bring focused awareness as feelings surface.
- Refer to the Golden Ray meditation, guided imagery or heart meditation.
- Check in with the client about any feelings that might arise from tuning into the pelvic floor which holds many emotions.

Mirroring: Moving Mindful Meditation

This activity is done in pairs and is an opportunity to practice sensing and tuning in to oneself and another person as a partner yoga activity.

Mirroring is a classic activity to demonstrate intuition. Even as an adult, I always am in wonder at the moment that the cognitive gives way to the intuitive and a dance of movement takes place between the two people.

There is always a moment of near panic as I stare at the person across from me, wondering who will be leader or follower. Moving in what appears to be molasses type slow motion, the activity finds its own life and takes over with a leaderless path. It is a way to practice mindfulness qualities in motion. One can practice letting go, beginner's mind and non-judgment in the exercise.

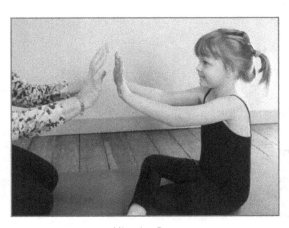

Mirroring Pose

Mirroring

This is a leaderless, physical activity that does not involve touch. The children work with partners and stand or sit facing one another. Instruct the children to place their hands 2 inches apart without touching. This is a moving meditation activity.

- Stand or sit and face one another.
- Both partners begin by placing their palms, fingertips to ceiling, opposite the other's palms 1-2 inches apart (right hand to the partner's left hand). The partners do not actually touch physically, but attune to each other.
- Practice being a mirror to one another's movements.
- Move slowly and simultaneously.
- Act as though you were looking in a mirror. One child may decide to move and the other person follows, then the other may lead.
- Use your senses, feel intuitively when to move or stop.
- Allow this to flow and change from leader to follower simultaneously.
- As one person moves, the other person will sense the next direction.
- Permit a flow to occur where at any time either partner can take the lead.
- Find a rhythm without words where both children mimic one another in a seamless way.
- Go gently from the cognitive to the intuitive.
- See if the kids can notice when they shift to moving together without separation.

This activity is a moving version of mindfulness. It is intuitive and comes from a different part of the brain than the cognitive. It teaches the children to let go, follow their intuitive selves and to have fun. The more one lets go into the leaderless activity the more the task flows with its own rhythm.

Noticing and Tracing Bones: Contents and Container

The Body Mind Centering principle of "contents and container" allows us to sense the outer structure of the bones and the inner organs. Bonnie Bainbridge Cohen in her book, *Sensing, Feeling and Action* (1993) explores the organ roll and states: "My experience has shown me that it is imbalances in the organs that underlie many problems that I see manifested in the skeleton, muscles and ligaments."

Tracing the bones involves touching the actual bone on ourselves so that we can feel where it is located, how hard, large or small the bones are.

Bones (Ribcage) as the Container

- Instruct the children to lie on their back or seated.

- Practice the three-part breath.

- Using fingertips, feel the size and density of the ribs and clavicle (collarbone).

- Notice how the bones move with breath.

- Notice how the ribcage is the container for the lungs.

- Pinch a rib lightly with the first finger and thumb, tracing with the fingertips the ribs from the sternum all the way around to the side and back of the body to the spine.

- Ask the children to notice how many ribs they can trace.

- Draw the ribcage. (Optional).

- Tap on the big bone of the sternum.

- Remember how the water balloon (container) held the water (contents).

- Discuss how the ribs (container) hold the lungs (contents.)

Organs as Contents (Organ Roll)

- Notice how the air goes in and out of the lungs and the abdomen.

- Roll to a side-lying position.

- Roll the body slightly more forward or facilitate this for the child. Holding the body slightly forward, but not yet prone, notice how the contents of the organs gently shift.

- Roll back very slowly from the 45° angle to side-lie again and slightly backward. Return to side-lie. Repeat this to sense the organs within.

- Notice how the organs "the contents" shift but are held in place by the bones "the container."

- If you are facilitating, place the hands over the child's lower back and abdomen.

What Do I Notice? Seeds of Mindfulness

This activity works on visual, memory, alertness, following directions, teamwork and attention, motor skills, somatic reactions and verbal skills.

Do it in either small or large groups or in pairs. This can be done in an individual session of therapist and student or in a classroom variation. The goals for this activity are:

- Engage in a quiet activity and feel somatic responses.

- Focus and observe awareness coming through the body.

- Notice wanting to move towards (attracted or reaching).

- Become aware of wanting to move away (pulling or retracting).

- Put your observation into a present moment response.

- Compare thoughts and feelings before after movement.

Mindful of My Reactions #1: Moving Towards or Away

- Look at pictures or a story that portray different emotional states: happy, sad, fearful, worried, safe, brave, light, and dark.

- Choose images of nature, objects, action, animals, or people.

- Invite children to say what they notice. (Colors, objects, etc.).

- Ask the students these questions:

  What do you see that you want to move towards? (Reach)

  What do you see that you feel neutral about?

  What do you see that you want to move away from? (Pull)

  How do I feel when I look at the picture?

- Invite students to take five deep breaths slowly inhaling and exhaling.

- Practice a yoga sequence: Warrior II, Triangle, Tree pose.

- Get on hands and knees. Do a crawl movement.

- Give directions for the Cat and Cow poses (See below).

Mindful of My Reactions #2: Moving Towards or Away

- Resume sitting.
- Ask the children to pretend that they are reaching for something.
- Pretend to pull away from something.
- Discuss which movement they like better.
- Discuss how the movements feel different in the body.

The Cat Pose

- Begin on hands and knees.
- Bow the head down, chin in towards the chest.
- Exhale into the pose.
- Round the back up into a dome shape the way a cat stretches.

The Cow Pose

- Inhale
- Let the chest sink in towards the floor, raising the chin up, let the head go back and look up.
- Repeat Cat and Cow five times slowly.

The Golden Ray Somatization

- Invite the children to stand. (You may wish to do this seated if needed).

- Begin the Golden Ray meditation.

- Sense your legs and feet.

- Place your hands on your hips.

- Feel the bones of the hips.

- Imagine and sense the hip bones connecting to the knees and the heels.

- Imagine a column of golden light going down through the top of the head, the spine, the legs, the feet, down into the center of the earth.

- Feel this sensation grounding the body as you yield into the earth.

- Take three deep breaths with this image.

Mindful of My Reactions #3: Body Cues and Feelings

Present the pictures from the earlier exercise:

- Invite the children to look at the pictures again.

- Ask the students: "Do you notice anything about the picture that you didn't see before? Where in your body do you feel or notice your reaction?

- Have any of your feelings changed?

- Notice if your mind feels quieter and your body more able to concentrate. "

- Discuss if the movement and the visualization helped.

- Focus on how you feel after these exercises.

Where in My Body is My Reaction?

Goal: Develop a body (somatic) sense for feeling drawn to something, a neutral feeling, or a sense of wanting to move away. For students to observe and learn when something does or doesn't feel right to them from information they receive from their own body cues.

1) Give the children a line drawing of a body with no facial features that fills the entire page from head to toe (it can be similar to a stick figure). You can invite the students to draw the heart, spine, pit of the belly (the gut) and the brain.

2) Use different color markers or pencils for this game. One color can be for feeling drawn towards, one for neutral and one for moving away.

3) Present a series of objects, pictures, foods etc. with different textures, colors, sensory inputs smells. Have the students sit in a circle where the objects will be placed. Use some pictures of topics that children or teens would have distinct reactions to such as: bullying, helping someone, littering, students ignoring someone, cliques, driving recklessly, animals etc. Allow for enough space for the kids to engage in movement. You may need to make some lines with chalk or string or indicate where the children can stand for the three states (feeling drawn to, neutral, or moving away).

4) Have the children physically move towards (reach), stay in place or move away from (pull) the object. Have the students notice where they feel a reaction in their body.

5) Instruct the students to draw on the stick figure drawing where they felt the reaction occurred in their own body. Have kids say or write down anything they observe about the feeling in their body and what picture it was related to. Have kids describe if they want to move towards it, stay neutral or move away. Ask the children to discuss where they feel this reaction was in their own body and what is it that they feel.

6) Instruct the kids to do the equal breath. Count out four beats for the length of the inhale. Then exhale to the count of four beats. Repeat his with five beats.

7) Practice several postures such as lunges, forward bends, back bends.

8) Discuss how our feelings are in the body and mind, and how doing the physical postures can quiet the mind especially when using the breath.

9) Review the drawings of where body reactions were located.

10) Discuss why and where the students marked reactions from their body on the stick figure pictures. Look again at the objects and see if anything has changed after yoga.

11) Do they have a calmer response (witnessing) or a more intense response (reacting) after doing the poses?

12) Be accepting of everyone's experience especially if any students feel resistance to the activity or unable to engage. Remember, we can learn from our resistance as well. Children who have experienced trauma may have difficulty experiencing a somatic response and may need more time.

Trace the Bones of the Foot

Tracing bones is done by feeling the bones with our fingers, and following the bone to where it begins and ends.

- Find the large and small bones of the foot without worrying about the names.

- Feel which ones are very big and very small.

- Move the foot and stretch the toes.

- Notice the different parts of the foot and how the bones move.

- Take the time to feel the bones of the foot.

- Stand up and walk around.

- Ask yourself which bones hit the floor first or second.

- Notice if the weight is on the left side or the right.

- Observe if your heel or toe side is more active.

- Sense if both legs feel the same when you walk

- Stop and trace the bones again.

- Notice if anything feels different

Shifting Weight

- Notice how your weight passes from the hip through the knee and foot.

- Observe how the weight hits the floor while you are standing.

- Standing, place your weight to the outer rim of the foot.

- Shift the weight to the inner side of the foot.

- Shift the weight to the heels and then to the toes.

- Move your attention to the outer rim and square the foot to have four sides

- Consider the foot as a square and feel the weight on all the sides. Go around as if it's a clock, toes, outer rim, heels, and the inner rim.

- Repeat this several times.

Tap the Bones for Quick Focus: The Sternum and the Manubrium

For a quick focusing activity, have the child tap on the manubrium, the broad upper part of the sternum. The sternum is the big bone that the ribs attach to on the front surface of the body. Start by finding the soft hollow part of the throat. Feel the manubrium, the bone at the top of the sternum at the level of the clavicle (the collar bone which is on top of the first rib). Children and adults will be amazed how hard this bone is. Tapping is also a way of awakening the senses because the thymus gland is in this area.

Tuning into the skeletal system is a simple activity to help children see how quickly the mind can cease from wandering. Each tap gives a proprioceptive jolt and wake up call to our mind and body. This allows us to feel the structure the bones provide us and come into the present moment. It supports our thoughts to become grounded through the sense of the layers of the bones. It can teach us to focus as we bring our awareness back to the large bones.

The Thymus and Boundaries

The thymus is part of a group of glands called the neuro-endocrine system which runs through the center of the body. This system separate yet similar to the energy of the chakra's is a subtle one but has a profound impact on the body. We can benefit from acknowledging the subtle existence of the two systems of chakras or energy centers and the glands which correspond near one another. These two systems can be helpful in understanding more about the emotional component of the yoga poses. The thymus, which defends against disease, is larger in childhood and involutes, or shrinks, at puberty. Linda Hartley, author of *Wisdom of the Body Moving* writes:

The thymus plays an important role in the body. As part of the lymphatic system, the thymus energetically helps create the sense of personal boundaries. The experience of loss of boundaries and protection often accompanies a breakdown of the immune system; stimulation of the thymus gland can help to strengthen the weakened boundaries and facilitate the transformation of fearful feeling into courageous action. It has a relationship to the adrenals, the center of instinctive courage. The thymus gives support to the shoulder joint and shoulder girdle and openness across the front of the chest. It moves the body forward and upward and the open posture itself expresses a courageous state of mind. (p.218)

We can all relate to courage and focus. It helps us to bring the mind back to the task at hand.

Tapping the Thymus

Placing your index and middle finger tips on the manubrium, tap gently but firmly on the hard bone, which overlies the thymus. Feel how your body responds to this activation.

You can also try walking while tapping. Sense your experience of courage and forward direction, the support through the shoulders and the openness of your chest. Allow your subtle feeling to develop as you practice this.

Back Bends, the Heart and Thymus

- The heart center is in the area around the thymus called *Anahata chakra*. A chakra is an energy center in the body. Back bends are about growing bigger and opening the heart. Benefits include: Opening the heart center and lungs.

- Toning the spine

- Energizing the body

- Waking up the nervous system

Combine the backbend with the thymus awareness of courage and openness.

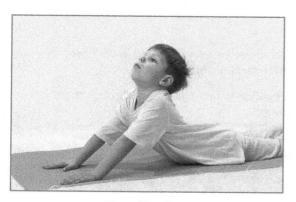
Upward Dog Pose

Upward-Facing Dog

When we do Upward Dog, we will take the support of this pose from deep in the pelvis, the organs, and up through the heart and lungs. Instead of pushing out with the heart, allow it to soften and rest yielding or allowing the arms to melt into the floor permits the body to rise as we reach with the head into the backbend and press up. Hold the arms straight and the chest and hips off the ground.

Tapping For a Sensory-Challenging Transition

Tapping the thymus can help focus students in a busy hallway or lunchroom.

- Can you be patient with your own body and its pace?

- Can you be patient with the pace the teacher wants you to walk?

For kids with sensory processing issues, being patient can be a challenge when they want things to happen faster or are uncomfortable in their own bodies. The bones can be used as a grounding tool, offering structure, and can help sensory kids to focus internally in a positive way.

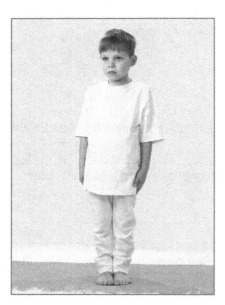

Mountain Pose

Mountain Pose: *Tadasana*

Tadasana, the Mountain pose is a quick line-up exercise before the children have to walk through halls to the lunchroom.

- Stand in Mountain pose

- Invite the student to stand tall as a mountain.

- Embrace the quality of effortlessness.

- Maintain the natural curves of the spine.

- Relax instead of striving.

- Allow your weight to yield down through the bones of the spine and pelvic halves into the ground and feel the support of the whole body.

- Stand quietly in *Tadasana*.

- Experience the awareness of the Witness (the part of us that is aware of ourselves being aware)

Script for Mountain Pose

- Stand tall as a mountain and find a place in your body that feels comfortable.

- Stand up with a feeling of lightness and ease, without stiffening.

- Relax into a place where you are balanced in your feet and your weight is evenly distributed.

- Allow a sense of melting to take the weight through the body into the ground.

- With a deep breath, raise your arms overhead, or you can leave your arms at your sides.

- Breathe gently and easily.

TIPS AND TAKE AWAYS

- Provide a structure of acceptance, trust and non-judgment when exploring the embodied activities.

- Hold each student's experience with the utmost gentleness and openness.

- Know that the embodied activities may activate feelings that are not on the surface.

- Be tolerant of all responses, resistance, silliness, or non-participation.

- It isn't beneficial to force any students to participate.

- Give clear structure and a safe option for those who don't wish to explore.

- Be kind to yourself as the instructor and patient with the students' reactions.

The embodied modalities and explorations have multidimensional benefits for students. Even the students who sit on the sidelines resistant will have an experience to feel that resistance in the body. For the students and teachers who embrace the embodied activities, the learning opportunities are vast. Embodied learning merges mindfulness, meditation, somatic experience, internal sensing, Pranayama and witnessing the mind and emotions. For trauma clients, it allows a "door in" to deep-seated emotions. To learn to connect what you feel in the body with what you sense in the mind and emotions is a powerful tool that can help adolescents make critical decisions. We owe it to our students to teach them these imperative skills.

CHAPTER 7

Meditation: Tools for Stilling the Mind

MEDITATIONS WITH EASE

Meditation is an activity of focusing. The focus can be directed to the breath, a word, the absence of sound or can occur when doing an activity with full involvement such as cooking, playing an instrument or creating. Meditation is being completely engaged in something to the point that we experience ourselves as being one with what we are concentrating on. When we sit quietly, with eyes closed and focus on the breath, our thoughts become less noticeable over time. We witness the thoughts passing in the mind. We become one with the breath and a quiet place within ourselves.

HOW MEDITATION HELPED ME WITH PAIN

I had a direct experience of how meditation calmed me when I was 32 years old and traveling in India. I had developed a severe case of rheumatoid arthritis; every joint of my body ached. Jolts of shooting pains were so painful. I was fortunate to have a chiropractor assist me with diet, supplements and adjustments. After treatment for one year it then subsided, and I was cured, never to have this again.

I completely changed to a vegetarian diet, and I followed a strict regimen and committed to a meditation and hatha yoga practice. My joints demanded frequent movement, and my mind was always thinking. When I started hatha yoga, I found my mind would quiet down even more. I adopted an easeful practice of meditation.

Each day, I arose at 3 AM to sit in a meditation cave (a darkened room). I meditated deeply in this still space. I practiced focusing on the breath, and witnessing the mind. I repeated a mantra with my breathing. A mantra is a set of words that have a positive vibration or powerful charge (See Chapter on Mantra). I repeated the mantra silently to myself. This helped me go deeper within to a quiet place that is pure awareness and timeless. Sometimes it would feel like I was drifting off to the edge of sleep.

In my meditation, I would see lights, images, colors, and unfamiliar scenes. Pictures, people, music and words flew by. I later learned this is the pure space of awareness, where there is no separation between the experience and the experiencer. There was only stillness and peacefulness. When I meditated deeply, I became very still inside. This would uplift me emotionally and give me strength and detachment from my physical pain.

THE FLYING DEODORANT: AN EXERCISE IN BEING THE WITNESS

One morning I was dressing to teach a seminar. I took off the top of my deodorant container, and suddenly the entire cake of the deodorant flew in the air. I stood there watching it fly up in an arc, and then travel down and land on the floor. I watched this as if it was happening in slow motion. I witnessed myself watching this happen and thinking that it was hilarious that my deodorant was flying. My next thought was, "Oh dear, what will I use now?" In that moment, I was a witness to my thoughts, feelings and experience. I was fully present emotionally, but had some sense of distance as though the incident were happening to someone else.

In this story about my flying deodorant, I demonstrate how we often practice being a witness and don't realize it. When we are watching thoughts pass in our mind, like clouds in the sky, we are witnessing our thoughts. This is the foundation for meditation.

I have applied the witness awareness in my therapy sessions with a child with sensory issues. I was fully present, engaging a child to maneuver through a soft tunnel and then to climb on a ball, repeating the sequence several times in a rhythmic flow. I was in the moment, involved playing, and present to her sensory response to an activity. Yet, I was able to stay detached enough to observe her experience, and myself so that I could determine what was needed next.

Giving children tools to be a witness to their thoughts and feelings at a young age is a precious gift, as these tools to manage and engage their minds and emotions will last a lifetime. Instead of a child feeling out of control when he experiences a strong emotion, he or she can learn to witness these emotions differently and regulate sensation.

It is very empowering for a child to look within for the source of a strong emotion instead of looking to an outside source for its cause. Looking within gives children a new way of understanding themselves. They can learn to notice the many nuances of emotion, the small up and down of hundreds of mild reactions and sensations that come and go in a day. Instead of suppressing emotion, children can sense a nuance, a slight awareness of feeling. Like adults, they can learn to experience changing emotional states throughout the day as small hills and valleys instead of big waves or torrents. They can learn to modulate sensory reactions appropriately and to notice irritability, anger or sadness surfacing. The relationship to the mind and body can be expressed through simple games and tools.

MIND BODY PRACTICES

Mind body practices allow children to gain access to a more integrated nervous system response. Therapists have shared with me that they have taught yoga to students who later used the poses when they felt upset. The children would go to the back of the classroom and do poses to self-calm. Those children now have a strategy that can be utilized anywhere. When children can be teachers to adults, or parents be teachers to children and bring awareness to the equation, we are on the right track to helping families.

When we practice a yogic breath, we are changing our nervous system from sympathetic to parasympathetic. In this way, the deep breathing from the belly can reduce stress and make major changes to our health and well-being. A child can be taught to breathe deeply at any early age.

I have worked with children while they watch a yoga DVD. Over time, they have learned to breathe deeply. If you enter the classroom and a yoga DVD is on, the children are either watching or doing the yoga poses. There is a sense of quiet and relaxation. It is remarkable, how simply watching the video, the music, the images and the soft voice of the instructor can so easily engage children into a state of relaxation. When the staff joins in as well and also does the poses and the guided imagery, the students calm down even more, creating stillness in the room. (See Chapter #3)

Start this exploration of learning to practice meditation by enhancing observation skills and building somatic awareness. The games help children and young adults to practice noticing, key to mindfulness. This lays the groundwork for the task of observing and witnessing the mind's thoughts. This builds the skills for future meditation practice for open-and closed-eyed meditation from a body-based awareness.

Gentle Breeze Meditation

- Sit quietly in a comfortable position and imagine a gentle breeze.
- Notice any thoughts you are having.
- Make a decision to let the thoughts pass just as a gentle breeze.
- Allow the thoughts without trying to stop them.
- Release each thought.
- Witness each thought as it comes up in the mind and let it go.
- Be accepting of yourself in this process.
- Breathe in and out.
- Place a finger under your nose to feel the breath come in and out.
- Focus on the breath.
- Focus back to your breath each time your mind wants to chase a thought.
- Bring it back gently to the breath.

MY FIRST MEDITATION EXPERIENCE

I can remember meeting a meditation teacher in San Francisco in 1974. There were about a thousand people in the room. People were standing in a long line, waiting to go up and spend a few minutes with the teacher. The energy of the room was electric with soft music, anticipation and excitement. I didn't know anything about meditation.

I can still remember the experience vividly. When I came up to the teacher, he made a loud grunting sound. The sound had such a strong impact on my mind that it completely knocked all thoughts out of me like a strong bolt of wind and my mind felt completely still. My mind stopped for a few minutes. He also laughed and I could feel his happiness deeply. There was so much love coming from him. I wanted to experience that stillness and love for myself. He seemed supremely happy, self-accepting and comfortable in his body. I began meditating after this.

At that time, mindfulness wasn't as familiar to most people as it is today. There was no Internet, magazine articles, DVD's or mainstream books written about meditation and yoga. Magazines didn't write about how to quiet the mind. Except for a rare esoteric bookstore, this information and experience weren't readily available. People learned about meditation and mindfulness from a meditation teacher. One witnessed one's own mind become quiet in the teachers' presence. The teacher's mind state was very still, and you became still sitting there, even just for a short while. By sitting and going into meditation, you learned to quiet and witness the mind. With practice you learned to create that stillness for yourself.

Creating stillness for myself taught me to slow myself down in the presence of children with processing issues. Once I was playing with Play Doh with a 4-year-old girl. I had allowed the moment to be in stillness, rather than chattering and striving. I realized that this was allowing her to be in a state of meditation in the depth of her play and concentration.

BEING A WITNESS TO YOUR THOUGHTS

Today there are many books and courses on these subjects, and public schools are using mindfulness, yoga and meditation because it has positive results. A study by Dr. John Medina, author of *Brain Rules*, comparing walking and yoga, proved that the increase in oxygen from yoga's deep breathing created an uptick in mental clarity and longer sustaining results. This resulted in a positive impact on academic success. Here are some stories that can easily demonstrate what it means to witness our thoughts.

THE CLOUD IN THE HOSPITAL

I had been meditating on and off for 5 years when I had to go to surgery for a repetitively dislocating shoulder. That evening, while lying quietly in the hospital bed, I was reflecting on my life. My mind, as always, was active. I was scared and concerned about the outcome of my surgery. As I attempted to sleep, I could see a white cloud of palpable loving energy hover above my body as I glided into meditation. I remember noticing and sensing its energy of peace and safety. It was clearly there to give me a message, and it comforted me as I fell asleep.

THE FLAG POLE

One morning in St. Louis, I was sitting in a Starbucks. There was a tremendous wind blowing outside shaking the glass wall where I was sitting. As I looked outside, I saw a flagpole and a flag blown every which way by the ferocious winds. I sat quietly with my warm coffee inside the building and witnessed the wind blowing. The flag moved around wildly. It occurred to me that the flag was very much like the mind. The flag was attached to the pole and it didn't blow away, it just blew around uncontrollably. I thought of this analogy:

- The wind is like our thoughts or our reactions to outer events that constantly blow the mind here and there emotionally.
- The flag is like our mind, responding to thoughts as the wind blows.
- The pole is the breath, grounding us.
- The halyard tethers the flag (the mind) to the pole(the breath)
- When the mind (flag) is tethered to the pole (the breath), it hangs on despite being blown around by heavy winds.
- The halyard is our choice or will to hold on to the breath.

Home Plate and Please Don't Run the Bases Meditation

This is an excellent guided imagery for children who love baseball and sports:

- Sit quietly and breathe in and out at "home plate."
- Watch the thoughts passing as you would watch a ball being pitched.
- Allow the breath to be "home plate."
- Hold your focus on inhale and exhale.
- Gently nudge the mind back to "home plate" when it wants to run the bases.
- Encourage the mind to just let thoughts pass by.
- Focus back to the breath "home plate" rather than follow the thoughts (Run the bases)

The Flying Car

- Imagine riding in an open car through the sky.
- See yourself laughing and having fun.
- Hold on tight to keep from falling.
- Feel the bumpy ride as you move up and down, left and right.
- Focus on the breath as you inhale and exhale.
- Imagine the car is your breath keeping you safe.
- Hold tight to the car and let go of each thought as it arises.
- Watch the thoughts pass into the distance just as the objects you see below pass away as you drive by.
- Enjoy sitting in the stillness as you go deeper on the journey.

TIPS AND TAKE AWAYS

1. Remember that practicing witnessing is much easier for children than adults, because children are so close to the present moment.

2. Take a moment to notice your own breathing, settle down and establish yourself in a calm state before starting the activities.

3. If time is limited, just sit quietly and do a simple guided imagery of a cloud passing, Golden Ray with deep breathing or The Flying Car, equal breath.

4. Use the somatic and embody cues readily.

5. Let the kids describe their meditation experiences.

6. Try to follow the kids' lead and honor their intuitive experience.

7. As you shift into this new awareness, remember to be as gentle with yourself and the children as you would be holding a baby bird.

8. Allow whatever comes up for the children to be part of the activity, holding a safe space that is large enough for even a few exaggerated tales or giggles.

Learning to meditate is a cumulative process, and every time you invest a few minutes you are building your bank of meditation practice. It is like riding a bike; once you have felt it you will be able to return to that awareness with little effort.

Understanding the concept of the witness, watching and observing our thoughts helps us to allow our mind to quiet down. In meditation, the goal isn't to have fewer thoughts or to stop thinking, it is to take a dip into the deep reserves of stillness and rejuvenation that is accessible to everyone within ourselves. By focusing on the breath, we are able to shift to a state of pure awareness, and we experience the mind becoming quiet. Be patient with this developing practice and honor every experience, as there isn't any right or wrong. Open-eyed meditation while focusing on the breath brings us to the same awareness. Becoming deeply focused in an activity such as drawing, dancing, cooking, skateboarding or many other tasks that involve focusing can also bring the same quiet awareness or by repeating a positive thought or a mantra. It can also increase the ability to concentrate, remember and develop compassion.

CHAPTER 8

Yoga Philosophy and Contemplation in Every Day Life

YAMAS AND NIYAMAS

In yoga, the *Yamas* and *Niyamas* from Patanjali's *Yoga Sutras*, give us important constructs for daily living. The Yamas (called ethical restraints) and the *Niyamas* (lifestyle observances) are part of the eight limbs of yoga. The remaining 6 limbs, are: *Asana*–posture, *Pranayama*–breathing, *Pratyahara*–withdrawal of the senses, *Dharana*–one pointed focus, *Dhyana*–meditation, and *Samadhi*–oneness.

I have chosen to focus on the the *Yamas* and *Niyamas* because they can be easily applied to family life and school. Helping us to do non-harm (*Ahimsa*) can be a program for anti-bullying. Non-grasping (*Aparigraha*) can be an antidote to our consumer culture.

We need to empower children in an experiential way, so they "get it " in the body to counter the negative onslaught of the stress of modern life. Where we used to play outside we now use iPads on the couch. We used to play musical instruments and now we listen passively to iTunes®. We used to ride bicycles, hike and climb trees, and now due to safety concerns kids aren't allowed to play outside without supervision. Parents struggle with childcare and jobs, and a simple activity of going to the park after school has to be scheduled. Every day, our hurried, complicated, and sedentary lives take us further and further away from the experience of a natural integration of body and mind.

Electronics can become the only connection to the world for some children. Yet this passive activity needs to be consciously balanced with other activities. Unless we make an effort to do this, we are doing our children and selves a disservice. Our children need us as adults to create and sustain that mind-body integration which is felt when walking in nature, playing a musical instrument or actively listening. It is experienced in arts, sports, or contemplation. These are the experiences that take us out of ourselves. Without these types of activities, our children may be missing a significant aspect of childhood and learning. We even may be shortcutting the human experience. Yet, through yoga, meditation, the arts, movement and lifestyle choices, we have a door back in. Unless we open this door, a sense of having a healthy, fully enlivened lifestyle, ripe with learning potential for ourselves and our children, could easily slip from our grasp.

SUPPORT TO FAMILIES AND TEACHERS: YAMAS AND NIYAMAS

I have chosen to focus on the specific principles of the *Yamas* (ethical restraints)and *Niyamas* (lifestyle observances) that can be applied immediately into our life and classroom. Examples such as not- bullying, truthfulness, not-stealing, keeping clean and uncluttered are relevant for our lives. Joan Shivarpita Harrigan, a practicing psychologist and the director of Patanjali Kundalini Yoga Care, states why they are worth looking at: "It contains essential advice for daily living. Patanjali has offered us guidelines that will allow us to have enhanced emotional and mental well-being and a more fulfilling and meaningful life. The *Yoga Sutra* is specifically designed to lead to greater happiness and spiritual fulfillment for you and everyone around you."

Team Building and Yoga Values

Partner yoga can be used for teaching team skills and dialogue. In mirroring, Back-to-back breathing, standing or sitting holding your partner's hands, or supporting each other during balance poses, is an opportunity to practice the qualities of *Yamas* and *Niyamas*. Partner yoga visits the qualities of listening, sharing, taking turns, and connecting. It is having a dialogue with the body and also teaches us not be attached to letting-go and beginning again. These are important qualities for work as a team and on a job. It embodies mindfulness qualities of beginner's mind and patience.

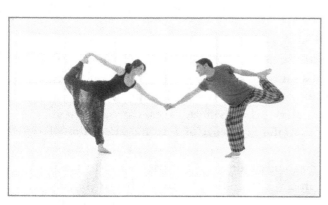

Suspension Bridge Pose

Suspension Bridge

- Find a partner who is about the same size.
- Begin practicing breathing in and out.
- Try to get your breathing in sync with one another.
- Hold your arm out and grasp each other's hand with one arm for support.
- Standing on one leg, raise the other leg behind, bending the knee as you grasp the foot with your other hand.
- Maintain your balance supporting one another.
- Continue to hold each other's hand and come again slowly to stand.

The Arch

- Sit opposite your partner on the floor.
- Observe your breath going in and out.
- Sit on the floor with knees bent and feet under your knees.
- Reach out with arms extended and grasp the arms of your partner.
- Hold your partner securely.
- Raise one foot up at a time, and place it touching the foot of your partner.
- Holding the arms secure, make an arch with the legs as you bring the other foot up to touch your partner's foot.
- Balance with legs raised and feet touching.

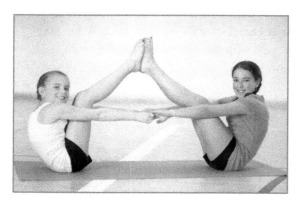

The Arch Pose

Values Index Cards: *Yama* **and** *Niyama*

Write one of the qualities from the *Yama*, *Niyama* list on an index card, blackboard or smart board. The cards can be used in the classroom as:

- The thought for the day

- The principle to practice for the week, day or hour

- A refocusing quality when having a difficult time

- For discussion about that quality in the children's lives

Ask Questions About the Qualities

- How can I practice this in my life at school and home?

- Is there anyone close to me that I can help practice this quality?

- Do I need more or less of this quality?

- When did the opposite of this quality happen?

- When is it the most important for me to practice this quality?

DEFINING THE *YAMAS* FOR DAILY LIFE

- *Ahimsa:* <u>Non-violence</u>. This can refer to not thinking thoughts and taking actions that are hurtful or violent, choosing to not indulge in violent games, speech, thoughts or actions or doing hurtful things. Do no harm and let things be

- *Satya:* <u>Truthfulness</u>. This can refer to sitting quietly and listening to your feelings, and tuning in when you speak to communicate what is true and helpful to others.

- *Asteya:* <u>Non-Stealing</u>: This refers to not using up or wasting others' time and energy for yourself and also literally not stealing.

- *Brahmacharya:* <u>Energy Moderation</u>. This refers to knowing when to use your energy to rest or be active, or when to walk away and avoid a conflict. It can refer to knowing when to stop listening to a friend repeating the same story over again, and choosing instead to do your homework or chores. It can refer to knowing when not to chase after every desire or pursue a desire that may not be helpful in the long term.

- *Aparigraha:* <u>Non-clinging, non-grasping</u>. This quality is useful in letting go of what isn't really yours, or not holding onto a bad experience too long, not keeping it alive when you can dismiss it. It also refers to not needing every new type of product that comes out, not clinging to friends or sad stories that aren't good for you in the long run. It can also refer to letting go of desiring something that you didn't get, and moving on. This can refer to not identifying with a feeling that you have to have something just because it makes you happy, ("I must have that chocolate ice cream. ") Also, not being overly attached to a positive experience if it may be distracting you from being in the present moment (thinking too much about a past event, e. g.,. a movie you liked, or your friend's new phone, when it's time to move on to other things). It is about being in the current moment and not needing more.

Defining the *Niyamas*

Saucha: Purity. Refers to keeping things clean and orderly.

Santosha: Contentment. Being happy in the present moment with what you have and where you are.

Tapas: Right effort: This refers to your willingness and possible discomfort in doing the hard work that it takes to accomplish your goal, to go through a difficult passage or endure with self-discipline. It can refer to hanging in on a group project when your group isn't working well together, and persevering until everyone gets it right, practicing a musical instrument or a project that appears difficult, and working through the feelings of fear or inadequacy to reach completion.

Swadhaya: Self-study. This refers to doing self-inquiry and looking within for our happiness, instead of outside. It refers to asking ourselves, "Who am I and how do I live? Do I leave my homework until the last minute? Do I tend to make good choices? Do I treat others with respect?"

Ishvara Pranidhana: Dedication to the highest: This refers to looking for the highest good in every moment and letting that guide you.

What is Attunement?

A definition of attunement from Merriam Webster® is: to cause (a person, company, etc.) to have a better understanding of what is needed or wanted by a particular person or group, to bring into harmony, tune to, make aware or responsive. When I think of the word attunement, I can't help but remember my daughter's elementary school string orchestra of cellos and violins. The loving focus and inner stillness of the music teacher was palpable as he went from student to student tuning the instruments. His compassion, patience and acceptance of what was in front of him, was mesmerizing and would infuse the room. The parents patiently waited in the audience, listening to the cacophony of sound. They talked softly and watched in fascination. It was as if they were somatically experiencing the instruments being tuned. The music director would step forward to give the audience a signal that he had finished this finely crafted task. I felt a sense of alertness and anticipation as the parents listened. The children could now produce a piece of music worth listening to. I felt a sense of ease and peace. I sensed in the room that all was well in that moment.

In the same way a music teacher tunes the instruments, giving support to the students to do their job well, a family can tune their lives to give support to one another. The parents may need help to learn to do this. Therapists can offer tools based on embodying, mindfulness, and breathing to teach parents. This support cuts across cultures, religions, race, and is based on yogic principles and the wisdom of the ages.

The stress of our fast-paced lives increases the risk of losing the opportunity to "attune" again to what is important to us. Having a holistic profile offers us a framework and a door to find our way back again to what's important and of personal value. We can see our reactions to what is out of our control and is causing stress. When we make a choice to hold the stress differently, empowering the whole family, it becomes much easier to let go of non-supportive, negative habits.

The Attunement Profile: Cultivating Balance Helps Therapists and Families

In the 30 years I have worked with children and families, I have learned that we are never just treating the child in a vacuum. As I travel around the country, I have heard that many school therapists consult with parents and teachers and have reduced treatment time with children. Therapists are often instructing the parents to deliver the treatment to a child.

I would encounter a myriad of parental issues including finances, divorce, kids' behaviors, nutrition, family dynamics and childcare. I would meet parents trying to raise children without a guidebook for parenting or their own personal fulfillment. As a consultant, I wanted to give clients options to their stressful lifestyle in a non-judgmental way. I asked questions such as:

- Would you enjoy having a family discussion?
- Would you enjoy having a connection to something greater than yourself?
- Would you enjoy making time for silence?

As a consultant therapist working with families, I struggled to find any adequate holistic assessments, so I developed my own. I felt if we could examine family life in terms of mind, body, and spirit, we could better help our kids and ourselves. I gleaned from my own life experience, as a meditator, a Waldorf parent, an occupational therapist and the single mother of an adopted child, and I designed the questions to help others cultivate balance. I used visual images with questions.

Families today are finding it more difficult with work and after school activities to have dinners with everyone in the family together and it is becoming a lost art. A question on the profile might be: Does the schedule of the family allow everyone to enjoy having a family dinner at some time? If not what would need to be organized so everyone could eat together on occasion?

I found and utilized an integrative assessment developed by Dr. Rob Ivker, an integrative physician called "The Fully Alive Questionnaire," which was divided into mind, body, and spirit. As I worked on developing my profile I realized that I felt that the mind, body, spirit were the keys to helping families come back into alignment from the myriad of stress we encounter. When a family would make an attempt to keep mind, body, spirit in balance, whether it was eating breakfast together, taking a walk together or all reading and discussing homework in the dining room, there was a better chance of communication, alleviating stress and the child's improving.

Over the years, I have found that most families want the same basic things. Some of us have more recourses and capabilities. The mind body spirit approach gently presents many "doors in" to reflect, on less stressful lifestyles.

Letting Go and Allowing

I found in my own life that when I was over-stressed, I would at times perceive my child's behavior as the cause of my stress instead of the other way around. I would become short-tempered and start blaming. When I could take a minute to repeat a mantra or breathe, I could see what was really causing me distress. I then would ask my daughter to sit down and we would discuss the situation. This discussion would allow me to trust that there could be a solution yet unknown to me, ask for guidance and let go to a higher power. I often ask myself the question from the profile "do you have a connection to something greater than yourself?"

A humorous incident involving a flat screen TV, is an example of this question and how it plays out in daily life. My daughter wanted to make a particular room in the house into a media room and buy a flat screen TV. Given that I have never been a TV person, it was not easy getting onboard with her desire. She was all ready to strip a favorite sitting room of mine of furniture and create her media cave. Feeling pressured with too much on my plate, I expressed I wanted the sitting room as it was and set my boundaries. Secretly, I wished she would just let go of this idea.

Determined to fulfill her desire, my daughter decided to buy the TV herself, but asked me to come along. Giving up my anger and relaxing into the unknown, we had fun picturing a really cool media room, and seeing ourselves watching movies and laughing as we drove to the mall. At the store, I watched in awe as my daughter sat on the floor in front of each flat screen assessing which was the perfect one. She was very focused and motivated and arrived at her choice after discussing many electronic details with the salesperson.

On the drive back home, laughing and talking, she continued to picture how she wanted the media room to look and the type of furniture she wanted. As we approached our house, we saw a neighbor putting out a couch in great condition on the street. We decided to look at it. My neighbor's husband came out and offered to put the couch into his pickup truck and help us bring it into the house. We had a hilarious adventure getting it up the stairs. Laughing hysterically, we got stuck holding the couch on the steps and couldn't move. Then suddenly a solution arose and the couch made it up the steps. Voila! A media room was created.

I am always amazed at how quickly the universe can provide when we know what we want, as evidenced by my daughter's clear desire for the TV. When our thoughts are positive and focused, things happen. When I was able to get past my resistance, my energy shifted to allowing an unknown solution to emerge rather than blocking it. This has been a helpful technique when working with special needs children.

An example of this occurred when attempting to do feeding with a resistant child who didn't want to hold a spoon although physically capable of it. Although I wanted to follow his lead, I often fell prey to becoming pushy and wanting what I wanted when I wanted it. When I was able to let go of my need, he would surprisingly grab the spoon and bring it towards his mouth. The more I practice letting go of my resistance; it becomes clear to me that a hitherto unknown solution can arise.

Often, as parents, we don't understand how the stress of the life we are living is a factor in our child's behavior. We see the problem as outside ourselves. A never-ending cycle occurs as parents are stressed by a child's behavior and then the child is stressed by the parent's reaction to that behavior. Dealing with our own stress is paramount to finding some viable solution for the family as a whole.

CONTEMPLATION: AN ANCHOR FOR THE UNKNOWN

We create a lifestyle from what our families and cultures have taught us. It might be what popular culture tells us, or what society is asking of us. It might be what we imitate from others or have gleaned as important for ourselves. It might be the lack of knowing what else to do. This can have both positive and negative implications. No one really spells out what is the way to have a healthy lifestyle. There are many books about how to do A, B, C to make your children smart or creative. But we as a culture are failing miserably. Living life and raising children is not easy. There are many nooks, crannies, junctures, and all of it can challenge our capacity for patience, love and forgiveness daily. How we think and feel has the potential to influence everything about our health, children and extended family. Knowing how to practice contemplation has helped me many times in critical parenting junctures. Here is an example of how contemplation helped my family in a difficult time and was an anchor for me.

When my daughter was 20 she wanted to do service learning abroad. For months she sent in applications, applied for scholarships, and set her heart on going for the year to study abroad. She worked three jobs during the year and summer to raise the money to go. She was determined to do this. She received several prestigious scholarships. We kept meeting people who had traveled to her country of choice and had wonderful stories to share. She was glowing with the excitement. It felt as if everything was pointing to the trip.

One morning, a close family friend and mentor called me. He alerted me to a disturbing story in the news of a dangerous incident in the town my daughter would be living in abroad. He suggested that perhaps choosing a different country might be safer in the long run and better professionally. He thought that somehow this incident could be a lamppost for an opportunity to change the plan. Then the bottom began to drop out of the trip. One problem after another arose. Several long and stressful phone conversations with the organization around security issues occurred. I was trying to understand and sort out the details. I felt as if I was losing my mind at times. I was being torn between a normal concern about safety and not worrying.

I knew in my heart that the trip was wrong, and I was very scared. I was bracing myself for a difficult conversation with my daughter. I sat down with her to explain about the phone call from our family friend and what options she had. I told her she couldn't go under these circumstances. Of course, there were many tears and questions. She wasn't on board with my feelings and didn't want her trip to be deterred or listen to the family friend's advice.

What made the situation even more complex was that the organization we were working with didn't recognize my concerns for her safety. The next morning, I insisted that my daughter withdraw from the program. The program countered with a new safer placement by the afternoon and she was re-enrolled. I insisted that one semester was enough and she agreed. We went back and forth all summer, with the trip's departure date changing several times. It was very stressful. There would be positive conversations with the program director and then doubts as well.

Throughout all of this, I held dearly to my meditation practice. I used contemplation to feel my way and figure out the next step. There were days when I felt as if I were losing my mind. My heart and head weren't always lining up. I knew on one level the year placement wasn't right. Having made the change of location and reducing her time abroad to one semester seemed a better fit now. Yet something still didn't sit well with me about the organization we were dealing with. I contemplated, meditated and had serious conversations with my daughter and friends about the daily changes to the plans and trip schedule. There was a lot of pressure from the organization and the scholarship committee. It was very confusing to sort out.

Five days before her departure date in mid-September, my daughter came to talk to me. She had just learned from another student that the organization hadn't been telling her the truth about some important details. She was devastated, angry and defiant all at the same time. She wanted to go abroad, but was really disturbed that she had been lied to. We both felt concerned that important information was misrepresented to her. We sat quietly together in silence.

My daughter was raised with meditation and contemplation since she was a small child. Although she might not practice regularly, she knows how to turn within in times of crisis. She told me she was going to walk up a nearby mountain to contemplate what to do.

I sat down to meditate also. I wrote the problem out, and asked for guidance.

In the stillness, these words came to me: "drop it". I decided to listen and let go of worrying and also to let the trip go. When my daughter came in from her walk she told me she had contemplated and chanted (sang). Through her practices, it had become clear to her that this trip wasn't the right thing to do at this time. She was able to let it go with tears and open herself to the unknown of what would be next. She had come to her own resolution.

After a few deep breaths, we both quickly began thinking about the college where she was enrolled. She didn't want to lose the semester. The next day, with the help of her advisor, she registered for classes on the last possible day permitted. After much contemplation, she was later accepted in another study abroad program that was a much better fit for her. My daughter and I had truly used contemplation and other practices to create the right stepping stones and map for her journey.

I have used a three-step contemplation with coaching clients and have taught professionals to use it during my seminars. It has always created a powerful and meaningful experience for those who try it. Once, during a group coaching session, a therapist identified herself as being addicted to staying busy. She was able to realize after the contemplation practice that she needed to calm down. Such a simple awareness can be a monumental breakthrough.

Once I was teaching a seminar in the same city as a prestigious clinic, on the same topic as their specialty area. I was invited to tour and to present an in-service but due to time constraints we decided I would just do the tour. When I arrived at the clinic, I was greeted and asked if I would mind presenting a quick in-service. I was taken aback and started to breathe deeply to get in touch with what I wanted to do. I had about 15 minutes to spend with the therapists after the tour. I choose to teach the three-step contemplation. The therapists had a profound experience. They all fell deep into meditation. They thanked me for the deep tranquility they experienced. As they dipped within to a still awareness, they became refueled for the day ahead.

DROP INTO THE HEART CONTEMPLATION

This can be done sitting with eyes closed or open

1. Offer the practice with gratitude before you begin.

2. Write out on a piece of paper a problem or question that you have.

3. Sit quietly with eyes closed and focus on your breathing.

4. Sink into your heart, as you sense the heart area as a source of feelings while contemplating the question.

5. Focus on the breath and take several rounds of inhale and exhale.

6. Conclude your practice.

7. Write down whatever comes to you without censoring it.

8. Honor what has come from you as an answer to the problem.

THREE-STEP CONTEMPLATION

1. Offer the practice with gratitude before you begin.

   Write out the question or problem you would like an answer to.

2. Meditate with eyes closed. Use the equal or the three-part breath to assist you into meditation. Focus on the inhale and exhale, witnessing passing thoughts and letting the thoughts go. Continue to bring your attention back to the breath. Conclude your meditation and open your eyes.

3. Write down whatever comes to you from your inner self without censoring.

4. Honor the outpouring from your heart and inner self.

TIPS AND TAKE AWAYS

The teaching of the Yamas and Niyamas are a rich template to use for teenagers and for any age child. Take one guideline and explore it for yourself and watch the day through the eyes of that quality. Give yourself time and space to explore in your own way.

Yamas and Niyamas can be one of many foundations for how to live life and make choices. **We can call upon and apply these guidelines for teenagers and small children in social situations, family, life and school.** Through contemplation, we open ourselves to look at our lifestyle and where stress may be draining our lives. Asking ourselves a simple question such as, "do you practice self-discipline?" can help you to choose to stop eating cookies and get out for a walk with a friend or go to bed at a reasonable hour (See Chapter 14).

Contemplation can be done informally over a cup of tea or at your desk at work. We can invite our children to use these skills in critical junctures when decisions need to be made. Sitting formally for the three-step contemplation can bring remarkable results. It is a method of looking at our thought process and allowing our intuition to arise. When you use contemplation, try to avoid holding back from the activity. Just allow the thoughts to flow. As you become more comfortable, you will ease your way into using this helpful process.

CHAPTER 9

Mindfulness

THE CAMERA LENS OF DEVELOPING AWARENESS

When I was a child, I had a special book that began with a picture of an insect on a street. Then each consecutive page showed the insect as if you were looking at it from higher and higher up in the sky. The picture for each page was taken from a camera lens zooming out into a larger view from space. First you saw the street, town map, the county, the state and the country, all still showing the insect and the house smaller and smaller. The objects became smaller and smaller, and the picture reflected a view from higher into the sky. Finally, the view was from space, looking down on the continent, the earth, the other planets and galaxies. It then had pages with pictures from the camera lens zooming back in again and ended with the insect in normal size on the street. This book had a profound impact on me as a child. I would often ponder this concept of viewing the world from above and secretly loved zooming in and out in my daily perceptions. It also showed me the interconnectedness of all things. I didn't know that I was perhaps having my first exposure to developing awareness or consciousness, detachment or the witness, watching as the subject becomes smaller and merges into the larger whole yet never losing itself.

With the same understanding of stepping back and looking from a higher view at the whole picture, we begin to practice the awareness of the witness aspect of the mind. Then after we have looked with a broad view, we can come again to see the details from a fresh perspective.

The Camera Lens

Draw a picture of a person. Pretend you are looking at the person from higher and higher up in the sky. Notice how the person becomes smaller. You will be able to see a larger view the higher you go, the buildings, the town, and the continent. Pretend you are zooming out as the camera lens did in the story. Show the surroundings as you travel higher into the sky until the object you drew is very small. Take the pictures all the way until you are in the sky looking down upon earth. Then zoom back in. Try playing with this concept of observing your awareness, zooming in and out while you are observing life around you. You may want to write your findings and experiences.

CONTEMPLATING MINDFULNESS QUALITIES

While doing yoga poses, an academic lesson, or any of the exercises described in the book, you can contemplate a quality of mindfulness along with the task. Have the children either pick one quality for the class or a quality from the list below and use the mindfulness cards. Ask the children to write or speak about how that quality was present or absent while they did the lesson.

An example that a teacher or parent might say is the following: "We are learning a new lesson today in math. I would like the class to practice the quality of patience while we try to learn the new material. At the end of the lesson, I will give you a minute to share about your experience of patience during your math lesson. "

Define these words as follows:

Letting go: To release a thing or feeling.

Beginner's mind: A fresh, open approach, free of previous experience.

Non-Striving: Being where you are in a timeless way, and not trying to get to something else other than the moment you are in.

Non-Judgment: To not make a decision about a thought or action. To give up being critical, measuring to a standard or coming to a conclusion about a person, thought or action.

Trust: To have confidence in the reliability or honesty of a person, thing or experience.

Acceptance: Allowing things to be in the moment and finding a way of understanding about this for yourself.

Patience: Being in the moment and not trying to be somewhere else.

Gratitude: To be thankful for all that is.

Empathy: To feel another's feelings as if they were your own.

Mindfulness Cards

Using index cards, draw pictures and write the qualities of mindfulness listed above:

- Ask the children to help you define what the qualities mean.

- Look the words up in the dictionary.

- Use the words as spelling words.

- Explore: How can the qualities be helpful at home or school?

- Contemplate: Can you think of a time when have you practiced this quality or when you have needed it?

Mindful Walking

- Slowly walk around the room noticing how your foot hits the floor.

- Notice if it hits on the ball or heel.

- See if you can focus on the foot.

- Watch your thoughts as you do this exercise and witness whether any resistance to focusing on the body comes up.

- Notice how the body feels as you walk in this way rather than your regular hurried way of walking.

- Pay attention to every movement of the foot, leg, hips, and spine and then return the awareness to the feet.

- Be a witness if the body and mind offer resistance to this exercise.

- Try to pull the focus back into the awareness of your walking.

- Witness your thoughts and emotions and allow them to be part of the experience of the exercise.

- There is no right or wrong way of doing this exercise, and for some people the mind becomes very active during the walking.

- Use this opportunity to practice watching your thoughts.

- Write down in your notes what your mind did with this exercise.

Magic Walking: Walking With the Breath

- Focus on breathing with inhale and exhale.
- Try walking fast and then slow.
- Coordinate your breath with your walking.
- Try walking very slowly, almost in slow motion.
- Walk in a very straight line.
- Walk in a crooked line.
- Walk backwards.
- Walk with eyes closed and open, one eye closed, one open.
- Walk in a silent walk.
- Walk making noise by doing the humming bee breath.
- Notice what your mind is doing.
- Notice if you get bored and what happens when you get bored.
- Deepen your focus and bring the mind into deeper awareness of walking.
- Do the equal breath for the last few minutes of focused walking.
- Finish this activity with the Sponge pose.

Mindful Walking Dance

Have each child show his mindful walking in a slow moving dance performance. The children can add stops and starts, bends, reaches, moving yoga poses, mirroring while walking, animal imitations and sounds.

THE WITNESS AND INTUITION

Have you ever dropped something like an ice cream cone or your cell phone, and watched it fall as though it were moving in slow motion? What is the mind thinking when you can see something fall? Have you ever had the sense you are watching yourself, watch something? Who is watching your thoughts? In yoga, the watcher of these thoughts is called the witness.

Who is Watching

Purposely practice dropping a paper, a ball or a light object and watch yourself watching yourself. What is your experience? You may want to write it down.

Activities to Develop the Intuition: Listen Within

Can you think of a time when you had a subtle feeling and didn't listen to it? Can you think of a time when you did? The goal of the activities in this section is to help children and adolescents to develop the skill of listening to their intuition.

THE BEAN BURRITOS: HOW THE MIND CAN TRICK US

I was cooking one winter morning. I decided to make an old recipe and wasn't sure if I had the ingredients. I quickly looked, and found three tortillas. That would be enough for half the recipe. Looking in the refrigerator, I didn't see any other packages of flour tortillas. After I assembled the three burritos, there was a lot of filling left over. I had the thought that it was too bad I didn't have more flour tortillas. Then, a very faint feeling came to check the refrigerator for more tortillas. I dismissed it, as my logical mind said I hadn't seen them when I checked earlier. Later, as I was putting back the materials in the refrigerator, I opened the drawer for the wraps, and sure enough there had been another bag hidden, that I didn't see the first time. It was too late to use them now, but it would have been helpful if I had heeded my intuitive sense earlier.

Intuitive Exercise- I Have a hunch

1. Have you ever heard the faint and subtle feelings of the intuition?

2. Have you ever had a sense about something?

3. Did you listen or did you ignore it?

4. Can you think of a time when you had a subtle feeling and didn't listen to it?

5. Can you think of a time when you did?

6. You might want to write down your experience.

You Get my Vote. Develop the Skill of Listening

In this activity, students get to show that their attention is drawn to something by demonstrating a yoga pose as the response. Noticing what attracts your attention is the beginning of building the muscle of listening to our intuition.

Use the smart board, iPad, art, music, photography, advertisements or a lesson that you need to do. Ask the students to show you when they notice their attention intuitively being drawn to a particular thing. They can demonstrate a particular yoga pose such as Warrior to vote on it, or hit the board with the wand, raise a hand or make a noise or use whatever communication tool is available to them. To demonstrate that they don't feel attracted, they can give the thumbs-down, do a different pose such as Mountain, or do nothing and remain quiet.

THE TEA DRAWER

This story is about making an assumption based on what appear to be facts and finding out later that we are not correct. The mind tends to move in certain grooves and makes assumptions based on its former knowledge. Often these assumptions are incorrect.

In my kitchen, there is a drawer where the boxes of tea are kept. One morning the drawer wouldn't close. I was convinced that a tea box had fallen behind the drawer. My mind immediately jumped to the conclusion that someone hadn't been careful putting away the tea. I was ready to blame who I thought was not careful. Then I looked on the counter and saw the tea there. Letting go of my previous thought about the tea having fallen behind the drawer, I tried again and was able to close the drawer. Once I stopped thinking something had fallen and changed my assumption and negative thinking, I realized that there was nothing wrong with the drawer. I then could see my assumptions were incorrect, and how I had made an incorrect conclusion based on an incorrect assumption.

When we meditate there are many assumptions that may come up. We might assume that meditation is difficult, or assume that it is impossible for us to meditate. We have to keep reminding ourselves to witness the thoughts and not allow the mind to spin out on the assumptions. Often they are not true. Thoughts such as, "I'm not good at meditating" or "I can't meditate" or "nothing is happening" can get in the way of your staying in the present moment experience. For adults, teachers and therapists, these assumptions make it harder for you as the instructor to teach meditation to kids. Kids have such an easy time meditating. They are in the "here and now" and can just close their eyes, see, imagine and become quiet, easily. As an adult, you can better support the teaching of yoga if you can remain open and witness compassionately your own limiting thoughts and doubts as they surface and patiently let the thoughts go. Respect your resistance also and honor that as well. Stay with the resistance. Gently shift your focus without judgment. Try the equal breath, and you may find yourself breaking through to a delicious quiet space of tranquility and awareness.

WHAT DOES A SUBTLE SENSE OF THE INTUITION FEEL LIKE?

There was another big snow storm and the snow was piled high all around the driveway. The new plow service came late that evening and didn't know where to put all the snow. The helpful gentleman plowing offered to move one of the two parked cars for me. We juggled moving the cars so that he could plow each section. He then parked the white car near the open door of the old garage while finishing the driveway.

A few days later, I went out to the car to go shopping. I noticed the old garage door was still open. I don't usually pay attention to the old garage door. I didn't feel like getting out of the warm car and out into the cold again to close the door. Yet, there was a strong feeling, pulling on my attention to check it out. Without thinking, I jumped abruptly out of the car and walked toward the garage door almost as if something was propelling me.

As I pulled the garage door down, I glanced over at the white parked car. I then saw that the window of the car had been left open for the past 36 hours since the plow had come. There was snow inside the car. I thought to myself how lucky to have yielded to that sense guiding me to the garage door, or I would not have discovered that the car window was open. Quickly cleaning out the snow, I closed the window. If I hadn't heeded the inner call to my attention, the window might have stayed open for a long time and caused more damage.

Listening to our felt sense (intuition) or having a feeling about something is a bit like this car window scenario. When you are sitting inside the car, you can't accurately perceive what is happening outside and you observe from a logical place. To fully understand the situation, engage all the senses, tap into your gut sense and get the perspective from all sides that includes the intuition you may have to get out of the car or out of the box of linear thinking and open to what may appear illogical). Then you can have all your senses accessible (both the intuitive and the logical).

When Something Pulls on Your Attention

- Remember a time when your intuition was present.
- What were your thoughts, and sensations?
- What did you notice?
- You may wish to write it down.
- How do you feel when you listen to the small sense or voice inside?

Intuitive Spiderman (or Favorite Superhero) Game

- One child stands with his back to the rest of group. He is Spiderman.

- 10- 20 feet away the children line up horizontally as messengers.

- Each child holds a small paper with a message.

- Kids try to walk up silently without Spiderman noticing and place their paper within 2 feet of Spiderman on the floor.

- Spiderman can only catch you if you are moving.

- The messenger is safe when in a freeze position.

- Spiderman will look behind himself at the line to see who is moving when he feels intuitively he should do so.

- If Spiderman notices a messenger moving, that child returns to the starting line.

- The child who gets to place his paper unnoticed gets a turn as Spiderman.

How Does my Body and Mind Know and Feel?

What part of you as Spiderman gives you the clue to turn and notice others? Do the back and side of the body have the ability to sense movement? Does your peripheral vision give you the ability to sense movement? How can you sense the other children moving or nearby? How do you know when to move or be still so you aren't seen? How can you become more attuned to your senses and intuition? Does mindful walking help you walk silently?

BEING IN THE PRESENT MOMENT WITH MINDFULNESS IN SCHOOL

This story by yoga teacher Erin Kelly in her own words shows how using the qualities of mindfulness created a safe space for her students.

YOGA PROGRAM AT SCHOOL

The following is an experience of Erin Kelly a yoga teacher, "The library was an awesome space. The kids came in to the library at 11:00 AM. There were about 15 of them. I didn't make them participate, but they had to stay on their mats. A couple of them napped, but most participated. It took a few weeks to build trust, but we had fun.

"One day, about the fourth week, one of the kids chimed in, and out of the blue, said, 'I have never had a positive male role model, my brother is hooked on heroin and living on the streets and I don't know if he's dead or alive.' I was shocked. I was speechless and I hesitated before saying anything. All I could say was 'I'm sorry.' As soon as I said it, one student got up and hugged the boy. Soon after, another one and before long the whole group stood around and hugged him. One big group hug, some of the kids even cried.

"Later, I found out that this came as a complete surprise to every student. Nobody knew this about this boy. After class, I took the time to tell the principal. He was great. It turns out that he never had a positive male role model either. He approached the boy right away and told him that if he needed anything that it would be okay to call him, night or day. I was so impressed not only by the bravery of this boy, but by the willingness of the principal to help.

The whole experience was so powerful to me. It was such a privilege to be able to work with this group of kids. My focus was to get these kids thinking out the possibility that they can shape their lives and that their past does not define them. Many of the children lived in challenging circumstances: divorce, parents in jail, alcoholics, and poor families who were lacking resources. The kids were wonderful. We did a lot of affirmation work, meditation and breathing.

Quiet Time

The David Lynch Foundation addresses the issue of trauma in schools by creating a program called Quiet Time. Used since 2007 as a program to help at-risk schools and individual students, it helps children who live very stressful lives to alleviate stress and focus on learning by receiving the benefits of meditation or a quiet period of the day. The results have been outstanding in reducing detention and suspensions in many urban areas' roughest schools. It has been helpful in improving teacher retention, reducing children's stress and improving academic performance.

The program is administered on a school-wide basis. At the start of each day, there are 15 minutes allotted for "quiet time" that is used for meditation, reading or drawing, but not homework or digital devices. At the end of the day, the 15-minute quiet time is repeated. The children can only use this time in the ways outlined and there are no phones, iPad or homework done at that time. Teachers indicate the beginning of "quiet time" by ringing a bell. To learn more about this program please visit the David Lynch Foundation website to see more statistics and details about how to implement a program of this nature.

Creating "Quiet Time" Activity: Breaks in the Day

If your school is not able to embrace a school-wide "quiet time" here are some possible ways to use a similar concept and bring quiet interventions into the classroom.

- Utilize the smart board-Instead of the app with the busy noisy activities; find a way to watch an underwater scene, or nature activities that evoke a peaceful feeling (3-15 minutes).

- Start the day in your room with a short-guided imagery such as the raft. (See Chapter 3) (1-2 minutes).

- Put on a yoga DVD (10-20 minutes).

- Add yoga and meditation to circle time (See Chapter 7) (2-15 min). At the end of the day, include several minutes of quiet time. (2-15 min).

- Play Pandora® Radio classical, New Age, or instrumental music (1-5 minutes).

- Use music that is peaceful to indicate that it is a time to transition. Lead the children in the equal breath several times along with a standing Cat and Cow pose (Chapter 5).

TIPS AND TAKE AWAYS

Learning to be a witness of your own thoughts is a gentle process and requires self-acceptance as we struggle to do this successfully. It is so easy to not listen and dismiss our intuition. It takes practice to not react and quietly witness our thoughts and emotions. You can practice any of the mindfulness principles, such as non-judgment, patience, trust, letting-go, beginner's mind and acceptance as you go through the day. Invite the students to pick a quality. If the quality is trust, invite them to think of trust as they work.

Begin **exploring mindfulness with an open mind and heart**. It is about present moment awareness and can bring you as an instructor and the students many opportunities for growth. Whether it is an exercise in walking, breathing, or exploring contemplation, it is a process of tuning in to ourselves that brings results in self-awareness.

CHAPTER 10

Working Through Trauma with Yoga

BODY MEMORIES AND TRAUMA

When I was 16, my 18-year-old brother was killed as he walked along a train track on a college campus in the Midwest. For many years after this, the sound of a train, seeing a train track, the name of the college or the state where it occurred would be a trigger for me. It would send me back to the memory of our Rabbi at our front door crying as he delivered the news of the tragedy to our family. Within seconds of any of the triggers, I could somatically re-experience the trauma of feeling the disorientation, dissociation and nausea I felt in those moments of first hearing the heartbreaking news.

The shutting-down of all feelings and body sensation began later that evening when I was asked by my disoriented mother to call my brother's girlfriend Elle and tell her about my brother's death. Dutifully, and unconsciously, I completely turned off all feelings and made the call. As grace was with me, Elle's mother answered the phone. I relayed the sad news to her and she was able to buffer the news to her daughter. My own posttraumatic stress went unrecognized for years as therapy was not as accessible at that time. It wasn't until I began meditating, chanting and doing body work and talk therapies that I could get near processing this trauma.

Yoga was the first healing process that I was able to see tangible results from. At that time my experience of yoga was chanting and meditation and a few physical poses. I participated in chants or singing events. It was during the singing that I was able to have a healing, freeing the emotion from me on a somatic and cellular level. Trauma becomes lodged in the body tissues and, as I sang, I let it go from my heart, mind and body. We also sang every morning a song that had the same effect of freeing the emotions and I gradually healed. (See chapter on Sounding)

Healing Heart Meditation

- Place your hand on your heart. Begin to layer through the body of skin, fascia, bones and into the heart organ.
- Allow yourself to be still with yourself for a moment and filled with the heart's own vibration of love for yourself and others. Even if your mind is busy, put the thoughts on the imaginary shelf and focus on the breath.
- Breathing, bring to your mind's eye an image and thought of anything that evokes joy for you.
- Allow that joy to fill your being. Focus on the immediate feeling of joy as your heart leaps when you bring your beloved image to mind. It can be of nature, a friend, music, art, family or any image that speaks to you.
- It is this actual moment of remembrance of the joy that we are focusing on (such as seeing an old friend, tasting favorite food, relishing a beautiful color). This yogic technique comes from the ancient yoga scriptures that teach us how to connect with the universal consciousness of joy.
- Breathe with an inhale for 4 counts and hold the breath for 2 counts. Then allow a long exhale for 6 counts and hold again for 2 counts to empty the breath. Repeat this several times.

As we do this meditation we bring ourselves to the awareness that joy is our natural birthright and our inherent nature. As we connect to our deepest self, we find the strength to let go of pain.

Often as the body relaxes while doing the physical poses and the deep breathing in yoga, feelings may surface that are generally armored in the body–mind. **It is important to give space and be open to whatever may occur in a yoga session and neither judge nor hold to any routine that would shut down any client's emerging feelings. This is why we do Sponge pose (Savasana)** the relaxation pose at the end of a yoga session. We rest deeply after all the activity, integrating the experience nonverbally and meditating while we lie quietly. Also at the end of the session, it can be helpful to do a hand mudra that can be calming and comforting to seal in the practice. The activities below use hand mudras and poses to help heal trauma.

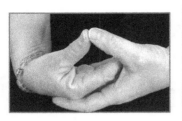

Calming Hand Mudra Pose

Calming Hand Mudra

In this hand position, called *Dhyana* mudra we cradle the right hand in the left hand on our lap and press gently the tips of the thumbs. This mudra is for contemplation and brings a sense of calm.

Tools Using Yoga for Trauma

The following suggested activities might be helpful for working with trauma:

- Deep breathing use the four-inhale, hold four, exhale six, hold two to empty (Chapter 5).

- Restorative poses. Do not hold poses for extended time as can trigger emotions. Only use for when appropriate for a few minutes.

- Guided imagery: The Anchor (Chapter 13).

- Guided imagery of meeting the friend (Chapter 3).

- Sensory corners and making cocoon-like environments with material, tents, pillows. (Chapter2).

- Gentle yoga.

- Using soft and relaxing music.

- Guided Meditations: Where in my body is my reaction (Chapter 6).

- Shift dissociation with grounding poses Warrior 2, tracing bones, ha breaths, guided imagery with embody cues (Chapter 6).

- Golden Ray meditation.

SOMATIC STRATEGIES FOR PARENTING: ACCESSING BOUNDARIES

I am traveling in China with my daughter who speaks Chinese. We are on an overnight train and it is almost time for our stop. The train attendant has come and is looking for our tickets. My daughter is holding our tickets and has gone for a walk with a friend she met, so I have no ticket. I don't speak any Chinese and the people around me speak no English.

The train is stopping 15 minutes earlier than the schedule, and we did not know this. In my best hand gestures, I indicate I will go look for my daughter who speaks Chinese and has the tickets. My anxiety level is very high, and I realize I am experiencing culture shock. Feeling abandoned, I greet my daughter with anger that is not helpful for the situation. She feels upset with my anxiety and blame. In reality, neither of us knew the train would stop early or intended to cause one another stress.

Later when we arrive at the hotel, I take a moment to calm myself with the breath. By breathing deeply, I am able to get in touch with my feelings of vulnerability and dependence because I don't know the language. I realize this trip is more stressful than I had anticipated. Before I speak, I ground myself using embody cues, finding my feet and yielding into the ground. I do the Mountain pose. I am able to see that I need some agreements about traveling.

I am able to communicate my feelings from a place of calm and truth with an open heart. I ask my daughter to share her feelings. After the discussion, we both feel we heard one another's concerns. By using yoga psychology, I am able to shift my anxious feelings and be a better listener so that my daughter can also express her concerns. After our talk, we take better care of one another and have a lot of fun on our trip.

EMBODIED COMMUNICATION: GETTING CLARITY ABOUT FEELINGS THROUGH CONNECTING TO THE BODY

When we experience a trigger that reignites loss of control, trauma, a moment of intense stress, an argument or a traumatic incident, we might feel disembodied, dissociated, nauseated or numb. We lose our sense of physical groundedness and mental clarity and the connection to ourselves. Here is a helpful strategy called "embodied communication." It helps us to find words and sort out the feelings of our experience somatically. It can be useful in parenting and many other situations.

Plant your feet on the floor. Breathe into your belly. Soften around the face and neck. You can remove your shoes and stand with your feet on the floor. Try these techniques, when your teen, tween or any age child is talking to you, and you feel challenged to set boundaries. When we soften and yield, we feel stronger within ourselves and communicate in a more relaxed and authentic way, making it easier for others to hear us.

Embodied Parenting with the Mind Body Spirit Connection

- Find the breath using equal, *Ujjayi* or three-part breath.
- Soften in the throat.
- Yield by letting go of the abdominal holding.
- Release stress with belly breathing.
- Soften in the stomach.
- Assume Mountain pose: Stand firm and ground with the feet.
- Use embody cues: Pay attention to the internal body sensations and make connections from:
  - Head to tail
  - Back, front and side bodies
- Utilize the grounding column guided imagery
- Acknowledge what you are feeling in the body
- Practice the Ha breath

SOMATIC STRATEGIES: FINDING BOUNDARIES WITH THE BONES GROUNDING

Establishing boundaries is a common challenge for people with trauma or when parenting. Especially when children are in the teen years, it may be hard to say no. These techniques can be applied in work settings or with family members. Once a young adult family member was in a foreign country and having a challenging roommate situation. We did the grounding yoga exercises together over Skype®. Any age person can do these yoga and embodied activities and benefit from them. The first step is to recognize that you feel you need to set boundaries.

For some people a sign that boundaries are needed is a feeling of hardening in the body, while also possibly feeling sick in the stomach or head, feeling like you are being bowled over and light-headed. Sometimes we think shutting down emotionally is a way of establishing boundaries, but more profound is to soften, yield, and love ourselves deeply. We will feel stronger and others will respect our boundaries.

One of the ways to get in touch with this is through the contents and container imagery developed in Body Mind Centering. The bones, such as the rib cage, are the container, and the organs are the contents. When you are having a confrontation finding the pelvic floor is helpful to giving us the boundary of the body as well as a grounding sense.

Feel the ribs by palpating the bones and tracing them all the way from the front to the back. If lying down, as you gently move from supine to side lie to prone notice the organs that are inside of the container of the ribs and how they move with the body and offer tone and support under the bones.

Techniques for Finding Boundaries and Structure

- Stand in Mountain pose.
- Plant your feet on the floor.
- Yield your feet down into the earth.
- Breathe into your belly.
- Soften around the face, neck and in the throat.
- Let go in the stomach.
- Remove your shoes if it helps to make the connection to the earth.
- Stand with your feet on the floor.
- Make eye contact.
- Find your breath and start to focus as it goes in and out.

Pay attention to the inside body sensations:

> Head and tail
>
> Back, front and side
>
> Yield into the earth

Paint the Sky-Pelvic Floor warm-up

Andrea Olsen, author of *Body Stories* inspired this shoulder and hip rotation activity.

Directions for the Therapist

For the Upper body

- Invite the participants to start in supine.
- Give directions to take an inhale.
- Pretend you have a paintbrush in your hand.
- As you inhale and raise your arm up from horizontal to vertical to alongside your head, paint with any color you want as you are moving your arm through the arc from floor up to sky.
- When the arm is vertical, circle the arm in the air for shoulder rotation, painting the sky any color you choose. Give directions to change colors, textures, and brushes to enhance mobility. Repeat the rotation in both directions. Repeat on the opposite side.

For the Lower body

- Repeat this activity with the legs.
- In supine, bring feet to the floor, close to the hips with the knees bent.
- Slightly lift the foot off the mat, maintaining the kneecap in a vertical position pointing towards the sky (vertical and up) and begin slowly rotating the hip in a circle.
- Keep the knees pointing to the sky. Be careful to not point the knee towards the head as in bicycle (common error) but vertically.

- Slowly moving, pretend that the knee has a paintbrush attached to it and paint the sky as you move the knee and hip in a circle. You can discuss painting a shape or the colors if you wish.
- Repeat several times and in both directions and on the opposite leg as well. Move slowly and deliberately, feeling the entire hip joint. You can repeat this for several repetitions as this is opening the hip and the pelvic floor.
- Give time for the experience of this exercise, it is worth the time as it releases the psoas muscle, and this also releases tension in the lower limbs.
- Move slowly and one can also use the image of a clock face if that is helpful and give directions to move to a certain time. Or just continue to move slowly and carefully giving adequate time for this very effective exercise for attaining relaxation. (See Chapter 6 on embodied activities and How Slow is Your Clock.)

TIPS AND TAKE AWAYS

Creating quiet interventions for *Pranayama*, embodied activities and simply quiet time for a classroom or clinic treatment can be informal or organized. Whether you have only a few minutes for breathing or short guided imagery or have a formal restorative yoga session planned, **give the activity your full attention and focus**.

Allow time for the client to transition out of the session and know that even a simple breathing activity can create a profound emotional shift. Be patient with yourself as the therapist, and trust the process as the clients step into the experience.

A somatic approach of using the breath, yoga, and embodied meditation will support transformation in the body and mind. By merely opening the door of exploring the relationship of the body and feelings through the somatic exercises in this chapter is a step towards healing in itself. As we try sounding, embodied communication, the contents and container and pelvic floor work we are opening to unlock the clients emotional issues which are lodged in the tissues of the body.

These activities take us beyond the cognitive into a cellular memory. This allows us to access the feelings and release them in the body and empowers us to heal. As we embrace the new understanding of body boundaries through direct experience, we gain new skills.

As the clinician, our **own state is so important** and sets the stage for our clients to be able to open to the teachings we are bringing. Remember to ground yourself with the breath and start your own practice. Working with embodied communication can be helpful to anyone, and using even the simplest activity of the three-part breath can be transformative for clients.

CHAPTER 11

Mantra

USING BREATH AND POSITIVE THOUGHTS

It is Sunday, and it's warm and sunny with a light breeze outside. My 14- year-old is moody, and I decide to give her some time to herself. After lunch, she wants to take the dogs for a walk and I agree. We pack a snack, water, dog treats and get the dogs in the car. We talk very little in the car today, and I'm looking forward to the physical exercise that will be great for both our spirits. I'm thrilled that she wants to get out in nature. I am glad I have given her enough positive nature experiences while growing up that she is choosing this to make herself feel good.

The dogs jump out and we start the steady climb up the 20-minute walk to the top of the pond. The wind is refreshing, and sun is warm on my face. The gurgling of a mountain stream catches my attention, my most favorite nature sound. The sound of the water skipping over the rocks fills my ears and blocks out all the other sound. Focused on the present moment, I revel in that awareness of just being happy. I am fully in all of my senses. The sunlight and the foliage draw me in as I take in the beauty of the woods. I find myself gliding out of my normal worry and stress. I am repeating the So-Ham mantra while I breathe and walk with my daughter. We are walking in silence and contented.

I would often suggest the hike if my daughter seemed moody and not interested in talking. Just walking silently was bonding and nourishing. I felt I could almost see the fuzzy confusing entangled mental activity of her adolescent mind silently being erased by nature. All I had to do was walk silently. Sometimes I would watch my breath and repeat a mantra while next to her quietly in between some quiet talk. Both of us would return in a better mood. As she became older, she would seek the silent solace of nature herself, jogging when she felt the need to sort out her feelings.

Silent Walking with So Ham Mantra: Open-Eyed Meditation

- Walk alongside the teen and remain silent.

- Watch your own breath and focus on the inhale and exhale.

- Use a mantra "So-Ham" or a positive intention thought such as, "I am one with everything in the universe. "Then inhale on Ham and exhale on the So. Say silently one syllable on the inhale and then the next on the exhale. (Some yoga teachers teach inhale on So and exhale on Ham.)

- You can use any positive intention thought.

- It isn't necessary to invite the teen to do this. If you are breathing in this way, you will bring a peaceful feeling to the walk together that is non-judgmental, accepting and still.

- Just be with the teen in a "non-striving" mode.

- Reflect on the mindfulness qualities of non-judgment, and acceptance.

- It isn't necessary to discuss with the teen what you are doing.

- The teen might want to know why you seem so happy. You can share about walking with the breath and mantra.

- Forcing a teen to do this activity won't be effective.

- When you are breathing and doing the mantra silently, you offer powerful support to the other people around you with your calm state.

How a Mantra Can Help Anxiety

Late for work on a busy Friday morning, I was standing in line for a muffin at the gas station. Suddenly realizing how many people were in front of me, I became anxious. I took a deep breath, unconsciously, and the mantra spontaneously began inside me. This calmed me down and gave me a focus.

A mantra can be any positive thought and from any background of your preference. When I pause and say a mantra, it is a conscious choice I use. The technique of saying a mantra quickly alerts me to shift focus to the breath and the intention of the statement. Within seconds I plummet into the powerful experience of deep breathing. I am repeating "So" on the inhale and "Ham" on the exhale. "*So Ham,*" means, "I am that" or "I am in relationship to the universal self, my deepest truth, or my own rhythm. " This helps me to connect to something greater than my small self or ego.

Creating a Personal Mantra

Through the ages mantras from ancient traditions have been used for protection, connecting to our highest spirit, for removing obstacles and for experiencing peace within us. We can also utilize the quality of "intention" to create a more personal mantra. An intention is a statement that is in the present tense and the action of the statement is considered already attained. "I flow with change."

A mantra can be a universal thought such as, "I am one with the source of all things." At times you might need one mantra for a situation and a few months later need another. "I am love" may work for you at one time and then during a difficult life change "I flow with change" might be a right fit for another time. For young children or adolescents simple statements such as, "I love myself ," "I am happy with myself ," "I can do this," "The sun shines on me," "I accept myself " or "I am pure awareness " are statements anyone can relate to.

Write a Mantra That Fits for You.

The purpose of creating a personal mantra and an intention statement is to have thoughts that we can resonate positively with. Use these tips to get started.

Start with a pronoun or noun_____ (I, We, My Heart, the Sun)

Add a verb_____ (love, accept, am, feel)

Complete the statement with a noun_____ and add an adverb_____ or an adjective or description.

I love and accept myself the way I am.

I remain calm in the face of adversity.

I accept change easily.

Everything happens for the best.

I honor the light within us all.

The sun always shines on me.

How to Teach Students About the Mantra

- Give examples of a mantra to choose from.

- Share the explanation from above paragraphs.

- Begin with *Pranayama* (equal breath, Ujjayi or three- part breath).

- Explain the three-step process and the quality of intention.

- Allow students to create their own mantra and write it on a card.

- Decorate the card and have the student make it personal.

- Practice the mantra silently with the breath for a few minutes.

- Add a hand mudra if you wish when practicing for focusing.

- Sit in an upright posture with your back straight.

- Repeat the mantra as you can, when in need and as a focus tool.

THE EGO: THE SMALL SELF VS. THE UNIVERSAL SELF

Walking with the dog, dressed casually without makeup, I pass a store and catch a glimpse of myself in the mirror. I'm not thrilled with what I see and tell myself that I look tired and washed out. I start identifying with thoughts, "I'm old, and I'm unattractive." In that moment, I'm beginning to feel bad about myself.

Yoga psychology is based on the ancient scriptures of Patanjali and his directives on how to still the mind. When the ego is at work, it is weaving a veil over our consciousness; deluding us into thinking we are nothing more than this physical body, these thoughts or feelings, or this circumstance. We easily buy into the ego's work. We lose touch with our true identity, the pure awareness or universal consciousness, a place of love and acceptance within us.

Our small self or ego is the part that is always thinking limiting thoughts such as "I'm not good enough, I'm not smart, and I'm too fat or tall" or the opposite thoughts such as: "I'm the smartest" or "I'm the best athlete." All day these types of thoughts loop through the mind. A positive aspect of our ego can give us strength, a personality, even confidence. I'm referring to the part of the ego that links us to limiting beliefs. We have been exploring how breathing technique, somatic exercises and yoga can help us reconnect to ourselves and combining this with a positive thought.

The challenge of reconnecting to ourselves begins with a process called identification. We lose our power as we identify our worth with limiting thoughts, "I'm not good enough," "I'm not smart" instead of just noticing the thought passing in the mind. Identification with the limited belief elevates it to become a gatekeeper to our state of happiness. The gatekeeper holds the door closed to an experience of the universal self. The more we entrain ourselves to the limited thoughts, the mind becomes like a path being carved out as we repeatedly tromp down the grass walking along the same spot. It is as if the mind unconsciously will slide over to the groove of the limited belief that we created, instead of trying new ways of thinking.

Thought Bubbles: I'm the Boss of My Thoughts, Body and Feelings:

In this activity, we notice how we feel in our body when we think limiting thoughts or expansive thoughts. You can make a stick figure drawing with two or three cartoon bubbles for the character's thoughts coming out of his head.

- On a piece of paper individually, or the white board in a group, make two columns.

- On the left side, write limiting thoughts.

- Make a list of thoughts the small self or ego likes to tell you such as "I'm not smart, I'm worthless, and I'm a failure."

- Try to notice how you feel in your body; notice your posture when you think these thoughts.

- On the right column change your thought to a positive one such as

  "I am connected to love and it exists inside of me."

  "Unconditional love dwells within me."

  "I am linked to the universal love in my heart."

- Assume the Mountain pose. Take three inhales and exhale.

- Assume the Warrior 2.

- Do the Ha breath orchestra

- Do the grounding column, and send the negative small self thoughts down into the earth. Pull up the positive ones from below and mix them together to create a positive experience.

- Notice how your body and mind changes with a positive thought combined with breathing and yoga.

Tips for Thought Bubbles Activity

- Create a very safe space and use humor.

- Give personal examples and stories to warm up the group.

- Adolescents might feel embarrassment and prefer to do this individually. You don't want a student to be vulnerable and reveal a limited thought and then be bullied or made fun of by others.

- Preschool children can relate the meaning of the limited belief with pictures of different size animals. The animals may think, "I'm too big" or "I'm too small, "I'm too smart" or "I'm not smart enough."

- School age children can relate to a story about a character that demonstrates a limited belief and overcomes the belief by accessing his inner strength.

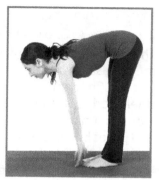

Half Forward Fold

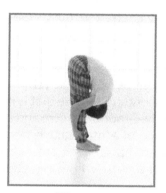

Uttanasana

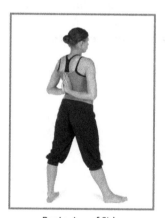

Beginning of Side
Stretch

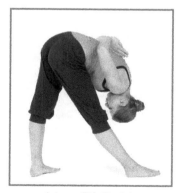

Intense Side Stretch
(*Parsvottanasana*)

Classroom Suggestions for Mantra and Yoga breaks

Half forward fold

Uttanasana

Beginning of side stretch

Intense side stretch (*Parsvottanasana*)

Forward Bend with Chair

Find ways to interject yoga breaks in transition between subjects. Remind the students to use their personal mantra for focusing or on one the teacher has chosen that fits the moment. Do a sequence: Warrior 2, Triangle, *Parsvottanasana* (side stretch)

- Practice silent walking for several minutes in the room.
- Do a short *Vinyasa* of Warrior 1,2, Happy Warrior
- Do the equal breath.
- Standing half-forward fold while sounding out the OH sound
- Practice *Uttanasana* or full fold
- Chair forward bend.
- Standing backbend with hands on the desk behind you.
- Cat and Cow in stand at the desk, with arms behind head.
- Do Golden Ray meditation.
- Do Gentle Breeze meditation.
- Do raft guided imagery.
- <u>Sitting in the Chair</u>: Begin to breathe in the three-part breath. Reaching both arms overhead take an inhale. Take an exhale as you move the arms down again. Repeat this five times.
- <u>Seated Cat and Cow</u>: Placing your hands behind your head and interlaced, do the Cat folding forward, bringing elbows together with an exhale. Then open the folded arms, bringing the arms back with a slightly arched back while inhaling. Repeat five sets
- <u>Side bends:</u> Inhale and raise the left arm. Lean to the right, with arm overhead. Exhale and bring the arm back to the center. Repeat with the right arm over the head, bending to the left side and then back to center.
- <u>Seated twist</u>: Find a comfortable seated posture facing forward. Turning to the right, bring the right arm behind you and hold the chair back. Continue rotating with the left hand, twisting the torso, and place the left hand on the outside of the right leg.

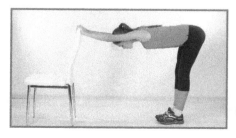

Forward Bend with Chair

TIPS AND TAKE AWAYS

A personal mantra is using the **power of a grouping of words with the breath**. The mantra has the intention to uplift us and bring us to a still, calm place within us. We take the words into our awareness on a cellular level of the body, by layering through our body systems into the tissues. Children and adolescents who have been exposed to trauma hold this trauma in the tissues of their body. When we repeat the mantra, combine the deep breathing, and posture, the positive thought construct of the mantra could be absorbed into the tissues of our body. The mantra repetition, *Pranayama* and poses become an embodying experience for the student.

There are many ways to have an experience of our own true nature. We can gently open the door to our deepest truth with nature, mantra, breath, contemplation, prayer, the arts and doing physical postures. Sometimes it feels as though we have to pry the door open because we are identifying so much with the limited beliefs. We may block an experience because the mind is so busy chattering. But as we get more comfortable tuning into the breath, the mind is coaxed more easily and quickly into a peaceful calm place. Once you are noticing the breath, the calming nature of the parasympathetic nervous system helps you to feel more relaxed. This is a powerful tool for a young person to have access to.

The **ego is the aspect of our mind that keeps us disconnected from our deepest self**. The deeper self, immune to mental chatter, physical pain or emotions, is a place of unconditional love that is in all of us. Unfortunately, our busy minds can block accessing that universal place. Meditation, mantra and breathing can be a tool. As we use a breathing technique and take the assistance of a mantra, we become less attached to the mind, emotions and body and go to a quieter place within that is in the present moment, and universally peaceful. We connect more seamlessly to ourselves and feel more whole and at peace. We can manage conflicts, stress and challenges more effectively.

When I use a mantra (or a thought with a high intention), it fills me with positive feelings. I find it helps relationships with others, because it allows me to tune in to myself, be non-judgmental, love myself, keep healthy boundaries and be more joyful. It helps me by providing a wedge between the constant chatter of my mind and its loop of worrying thoughts and to do lists. **Repeating a mantra keeps me in touch with my heart or my feelings**.

CHAPTER 12

Honoring Silence

MINDFULNESS AND SILENCE IN DAILY LIFE

As we become more comfortable with witnessing our thoughts, using a mantra and observing the breath as a focusing tool, we find ourselves enjoying silence as a quieting and rejuvenating activity. Silence can support deepening the experience of using a mantra and meditation . The activities below can be practiced to use silence in daily life.

Breathing and Silent Walking

While walking, practice watching your breath. After a short time, you will sense your breathing becoming deeper and your mind becoming stiller. This is a great time to repeat a mantra or focus on the breath coming in and out. This will deepen the relaxation and stillness inside and you will also notice more around you. Take note of how your senses are heightened naturally when you are focused on the breath.

A Silent Meal

Having a silent meal is an activity a family or class can do to experience a sense of quiet. You can decide to go into silence for a short time at home. You can invite family members to try this for 5-15 minutes or more. Keep a sense of humor about trying this. Do you remember the teenage brother in the movie, "Little Miss Sunshine," who refused to talk to his family and would only write on a notepad? This is not the kind of silent retreat I am referring to! Instead, it is a choice you make because you feel it will help you to calm down, self regulate and experience inner stillness. This activity is not to be used as a punishment for any child. It is not intended to give someone "the silent treatment" or used inappropriately. If you are doing a silent meal with family just make it fun, and see how long people can be quiet. The point is not to punish or reward but just to try being away from all the chatter inside and out.

Silent Retreat for a Parent

- Make clear boundaries with those around you when you will be on a silent retreat.

- Be sure to state clearly when you will start and when you will rejoin the family.

- Keep everyone informed about how they can get their needs met while you are being silent. This prevents your children from having a strong need to disturb you.

- Putting on a yoga DVD for the whole family to do together may also achieve the same results and help everyone quiet down.

- Do not punish or show anger at kids who can't manage your quiet time.

- Offer the family the name of someone who will be physically present as the person that is available to them in the house, instead of you.

- If necessary, you can arrange for the children to visit with a friend or play date so you can have an undisturbed time.

- Do not recluse yourself leaving the children alone without supervision or unsafe in the name of a silent retreat. Use common sense.

- Turn your cell phone off.

- Maintain a sense of humor as people try to talk to you.

- Don't be angry if you are disturbed; just witness yourself making an attempt to be silent.

- Accept if your children aren't able to give you this privacy and organize a better support for everyone to have their needs met.

- Practice contentment with the results, even if it is just a short time.

- The more adult support you can organize for the children spending time with others, the easier it is to be successful at the activity.

- Avoid using the silent retreat to escape parenting responsibilities.

- When the children are cared for appropriately, begin your retreat by engaging in positive self-care activities that are nurturing to you.

- Use the time to contemplate, write in your journal, do yoga poses, meditate, walk in nature and do *Pranayama* or watching your breath quietly.

- Do the drop into heart meditation or three-step contemplation.

Quiet time Indoors for Single Parents

If you are a single parent and want quiet time try these tips.

- To change the tone of the space, get down on the floor.
- Turn off the TV and find games or quiet activities.
- Play a game to see how long everyone can be silent.
- Listen to relaxing music together lying comfortably on the floor.
- Read books to the children or have them look at books.
- Read a book yourself and request they do the same.
- Use the restorative poses for yourself.
- Set up the children in a restorative pose.
- Watch and do a yoga video all together.
- Make food or bake together.
- Listen to quiet music on Pandora Radio° and rest on the floor.
- Play quiet games, color, do art while listening to music.
- Set the timer so they know when it's ok to talk to you in 3-15minutes maximum.
- Do not punish children who can't tolerate the quiet.
- Be patient, the more you introduce quiet time, the easier it will be for the children to participate.
- Habits don't change overnight, but practice is cumulative. The more times you practice quiet time, the easier it will be for the next time.

Quiet Outside Time

Set the tone that you are requesting the children play quietly and choose one or more of the following activities:

- Take a walk
- Go to a park
- Go for a ride in car
- Do people-watching
- Sit outside drawing
- Go to a café and read a book
- Go to a library
- Play at the beach
- Walk the dog
- Bicycle ride

Designating a time or place for silence, or a particular activity helps others orient and expect that routine. Whether we have experienced the quiet ambience in a library, a nap time at school or study hall, it can be created at home or in the classroom with simple guidelines.

Honoring silence in daily life can be as simple as turning off the radio and taking a moment to sit in the car and look at the sky on a busy highway and being fully present to that moment. It might be taking a minute to acknowledge the beauty of the day before heading indoors. When we allow ourselves to seek a silent activity either sitting or physically active, **we are giving ourselves a gift of a retreat** which is rejuvenating for the mind and body and empowers us in our daily lives for the next challenge.

CHAPTER 13

Sounding

BENEFITS OF SOUNDING

Sounding is used in yoga in the form of singing or chanting. It can be making a simple sound of OM to conclude exercises or used when we repeat a mantra. (a particular grouping of words that have a positive vibration). Luciano Bernardi, professor of internal medicine at the University of Pavia, Italy states: "The benefits of respiratory exercises to slow respiration in the practice of yoga have long been reported, and the mantra may have evolved as a simple device to slow respiration, improve concentration and induce calm" (Bernardi et al. , 2001).

Healing is impacted by sound in many ways. Mitchell Gaynor, author of *Sounds of Healing* (2000), and the director of medical oncology and integrative medicine at Strang-Cornell Cancer Prevention Center notes: "It alters cellular functions and biological systems, through entrainment, to function more homeo-statically; (and) it calms the mind and the body; affects the emotions, which influence neurotransmitters and neuropeptides, which in turn regulate the immune system."

Sounding is a way to use the voice and explore the different tones, high, low, loud or soft. You can also explore different organs and body parts by concentrating on the sounds of that area. Bonnie Bainbridge Cohen, author of *Sensing Feeling and Action* (says: "In order to vocalize, we must actively engage our organs. Without organic support we cannot utter a sound. The strength of our voice is based upon the degree of involvement of our total organ system. A blockage somewhere in our organs will be reflected in the quality and intensity of our voice. "(Cohen 2012 p. 38)

YOGA FOR SPECIAL NEEDS: MOVING WARM-UPS AND SOUNDING

I have found that severely multi-handicapped children respond well to mindfulness, gentle yoga and guided meditation in the classroom. Sounding out with a vowel is also helpful to aid in the relaxation exercise.

Sounding Session One

This guided meditation was used in a multi-handicapped classroom at a school for severely handicapped children ages 4-21. This classroom activity was also used with adolescents and ages 13-21 who had various diagnoses of autism, scoliosis, developmental delay, cerebral palsy, and were predominantly nonverbal. This activity can also be used with younger children and modified if needed. The program has one adult staff member to one or two students.

The Warm up Movements

- Place the students supine on their mats
- Invite the staff to join them on the mats, giving support in supine
- Play soft music from Pandora
- Invite everyone to participate in moving warm-ups from supine (5-7 minutes)
- Instruct the staff assist in moving the limbs of the students as needed
- Move one arm at a time inhaling up and exhaling down
- Repeat with the legs, moving one leg and then the other
- Do the same side of the body, one leg and arm, and contralateral, one leg and opposite arm.
- Accompany all movements with the breathing directions.
- Use " the paintbrush " "(pg. 95) bend and hold knee vertical and rotate hip
- Focus attention on the breath throughout the entire warm-ups
- Take 30 minutes in total or less can be adequate
- Plan for 5 minutes at beginning set up and 5 minutes at end for transition
- Do the guided imagery and warm up for 15- 20 minutes

The Auditory Sounding

The students did the sounding of "Oh" and "Ah" with me. Some children who normally have shallow breathing and have low volume in vocalizations sounded loudly and breathed deeply in our sessions.

- Lead the group to make the sounds by singing out the sound "O", "AH"
- Invite the staff to participate in the soundings along with the young adults.

The Guided Imagery " The Raft" from Chapter 3

- Begin a short guided imagery of floating on a raft
- Use Nature themes of the sun, air, wind, and sky
- Describe a sense of yielding into the earth, letting go and feeling as though you have no cares to assist the students to feel they are floating in the raft
- Remind with cues to focus on taking inhales and exhales throughout the session.

Connect-ed and Hand Mudra

- Instruct students to place the tongue on the roof of the mouth on a meridian
- Allow a moment to tune into a calm sense that is created
- Assume a hand mudra of two cupped hands with the left bottom palm holding the right palm and pressing the tips of thumbs together (pg. 76)
  This combination of the hands and the tongue is more advanced and complex.

Yoga and Sounding creates Social Skills

At one session, a student was invited to help with rolling up the mats during the cleanup. This student and I hadn't had much interaction previously, but I felt that the sounding had created a new relationship between us. She seemed to want to be around me and wasn't leaving my side and eagerly did the task given to her. Most of the room was quiet and not resuming its normal busy chatter. Everyone was deeply relaxed and quiet. I felt that the sounding for the nonverbal multi-handicapped students provided a deep relaxation experience. I have witnessed students have a similar experience when banging very hard on a drum during a music activity listening to very low tones.

Sounding Session Two

- We used **sounding and the three-part breath** throughout the activity.
- I made several "Ha" sounds and breaths out loud. (See Chapter 5).
- The students were lying supine, and so the proprioceptive pulling motion of the seated or standing "Ha" breath was not used.
- Instead, we focused on producing sounds. After inhaling, the group was instructed to exhale "Ha-ah. ". **The group demonstrated a series of sounding exhaling "Ah, Oh," and very low tones of "Ah."**

The Non- Verbal Students participated in Sounding

The students were making the sounds with me. Students who generally have limited lung capacity and/or volume, were able to **demonstrate a bigger exhale and volume** and make a **louder sound than usual** due to the exercise. Also some of the **non-verbal kids were making loud sounds. They seemed to enjoy the activity very much**. The sounding was continued for 3-5 minutes.

Leading the Sounding produced deep relaxation for the students

In the same way a music therapist sings and is a leader for a group, I led the group by sounding with full volume. Even if some of the students didn't continue to sound with me, being in the presence of my vocalizations had a transforming impact on the relaxation of the group. Everyone became still and quiet. The children ceased their extraneous movements, noises and anxiety during these sessions. They lay quietly on the mats. Being in the presence of the sounding was very profound for the students, and it had a calming effect. Sounding has a nurturing, primordial and ancient quality to it. Sounding appears to meet people where they are emotionally and have a comforting effect similar to that of drumming.

Therapist Instructions for Self–Exploration of Sounding

When a therapist or teacher instructs sounding in a classroom or clinic, begin to lead with sounds such as "Om" or "Ah." A tip for a practitioner, who wants to gain expertise with sounding, is to practice on your own. Once you begin to make the sounds yourself and explore how it feels in your own body, you will have your own experience. Your exploration will offer an understanding of the impact of sounding.

- Find a comfortable place in your body, either lying down or sitting.

- Focus on your breath with an inhale and exhale.

- Allow a sound to start in the throat with the exhale.

- Notice where the sounds start and then where it travels in the body.

- Allow yourself to try by hissing or making an "Ah" or "Oh" sound.

- Experiment with humming, making a low or high tone.

- Let the sound emanate out from deep within yourself.

- Experiment sounding with a fully throated expression.

- Remain in sync with the breathing and toning.

- Observe your experience.

Instructor Techniques for Sounding in a Yoga session
Students experience Sounding by:
- Listening to the instructor's voice as it sounds out, and taking that experience in through all the body systems, and on a cellular level
- Sounding/vocalizing along with the instructor

How to give the students the maximum benefits of Sounding
- Vocalize and sound out for at least a minimum of 2-5 minutes of your program. You want the students to get comfortable with the experience and also relax into hearing your voice. You can easily add more time if you wish
- Hold the sound vibration and vocalize it for the class, allowing the students to both listen and sound at the same time. Some students may choose to listen to the sound and take it into the body on the cellular level, and others will join in on making the sounds. Both are important experiences
- Honor everyone's choice to be there in his or her preferred way and there is no right or wrong

Your own emotional, meditative state and "open-heartedness" is your most powerful tool to communicate the yoga sounding experience to others. In the same way that we as therapists facilitate movement responses using our hands and have an impact on the student physically, the instructor's voice can have a profound impact on the student emotionally, mentally and physically. The use of the voice is not related to having a good singing voice. It is in the context of fully participating in offering these ancient tones through your voice to the class so that they can hear you and have their own experience of sounding. If you are working one to one or in a group, and there is resistance or discomfort to using sounding, a simple introduction to sounding is to try the "Ha" breath. Standing in a lunge position, or seated, raise the arms up and pull the arms down with the exhale while sounding out "Ha."

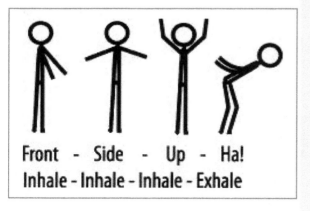

The Orchestra

The Orchestra
I call this activity the Orchestra because it reminds me of the arm movements of a conductor. The image of the conductor can be helpful as adolescents and children can easily visualize it. Conductor wands (paint sticks) can also be added for children to make it more fun. In the this version of the Orchestra Breath, developed by Amy Weintraub, called Breath of Joy, stand in *Tadasansa* or Mountain pose with arms in front. Raise the arms out to the sides, then up overhead while inhaling, and on the exhale pull the arms down and behind you making the "Ha" sound. Take one inhale for all three movements, moving the arms as shown in the illustration. As you bring down the arms and exhale make the sound "Ha!" loudly. This has both the proprioceptive movement of the arms and the vocal sounding and has a cathartic quality. It is a contained exercise that can be repeated.

Listening From the Cells Into the Organs
Sounding with "Ah" or "Om" in different tones brings participants into a deep state of stillness and relaxation. After the raft guided imagery, I often use the sounding tones. Sounding is like singing or chanting, only using a single sound and gently helps participants into meditation. Imagine one organ such as the lungs or stomach and you can send the sound into that organ. This gives a cue to the body of somatic awareness. Image all the cells of that body part taking in the sound.

Script for Explaining Sounding

"Find a comfortable place in your body and, if you wish, you may lie down. Gently focus on your breath with an inhale and exhale. I will be making some sounds now that will help guide you into meditation. These ancient sounds, common to all cultures, are from the foundation of all language. As you allow the mind and body to listen to the sounds fully, gently allow yourself to glide into meditation. Listen from the cells that make up the skin, bones, organs, muscles and all the body systems. While you perform this exercise practice beginner's mind and non-striving. Listen to these sounding tones fully with all of yourself and allow the sound to create a safe space in the room for you to relax."

Barbara's Experience Sounding with Autistic Young Adults

It fascinates me when I do the sounding how easily and profoundly the group will enter a deep state of relaxation. Often many students will appear to be sleeping or may actually fall asleep. The sounding takes the students beyond the mind and into stillness. When sounding, I take the sound of "Ah." I inhale deeply and, on the exhale, sound out in a normal tone "Ah-Ah" until all my breath has fully emptied. Then I allow a pause and allow the sound to float in the air. Then I repeat again slowly the sounding of "Ah.".

I also use "Oh" and also "Om" sometimes I vary the tones and go to a lower tone if I can. I may also use other references to organs and sound into the lungs, or the stomach. I do not talk during the sounding. I just allow for silence and the sound to fill the room. I repeat this about 10 times.

Warm-Ups

- Have the children begin lying supine.
- Instruct the students to move the head to the right side and then to the left. Repeat this several times.
- Instruct the students to move the arms flat along the floor from their sides and inhale and exhale.
- Move the arms up to the ears as if making snow angels.
- Move the arms from the side straight up toward the ceiling.
- Return the arms down with an inhale and exhale.
- Bring the arms up with an inhale.
- Bring the arms back down with an exhale.
- This can be done also with the equal breath by counting the duration of the inhale and having participants move their arms for 4 counts.
- Take 4 counts to move your arms from the floor to above your head and 4 counts to come back down.

Paintbrush

- Begin in supine.
- Instruct the students to raise their legs up and down.
- Practice equal breath 4 counts, then 5.
- Imagine a paintbrush on the knee.
- Point the kneecap to the ceiling as you rotate the hip.
- Rotate the hip and knee in a circle clockwise and then counter clockwise.

The Balloon

- Start with the raft imagery.
- Image a balloon in the raft.
- Fill the balloon with any worries, care, concerns, fears.
- Let the balloon go and watch it float up to the sky.

The Anchor

- Imagine floating in the raft.
- Imagine throwing an anchor off the raft.
- Watch it travel down into the bottom of lake and deep into the earth.
- The anchor sends grounding energy from the earth into your body.
- Send the golden light from our body down to the center of the earth.
- This grounds us whenever we feel overwhelmed.

TIPS AND TAKE AWAYS

• Inform the group that you will be demonstrating some ancient and universal sounds.

• **Make the sounds full throated and of adequate volume,** fully using the power of your exhale to create the sound vibration. Do not worry if your throat is unclear or your voice wavers as you start. Simply move past your own initial awareness of the sound, and it will develop into a solid sound vibration as you continue to make the sounding. You may experience your own body vibrate as you take the sound all the way to the end of the vocalization.

• Then inhale and start again using "Ah, Oh" or "Om" or other sounds. As you hold your exhale for as long as you can, and sound out, it invites others to feel comfortable and to try as well.

In my personal experience, the biggest challenge to sounding is to go beyond my own fear of being judged. The students and the staff would be in a deep state of relaxation and stillness. They would only be very grateful for the experience and thank me at the end for the session. After I cease sounding, I **pause and allow everyone to sit quietly**. I allow for the participants and staff to slowly open their eyes and transition back to the classroom or group. I **do not hurry the transition**. I have found that it is not necessary to speak, ask for feedback or give information at this time. Instead, I value the silent space that has been created. By allowing the students to remain fully present to their own silent experience and not hurrying the students out of the quiet, I am honoring the universal stillness within each of us. I aim to leave at least 5 minutes or more from the end of the sounding and guided imagery for the transition.

CHAPTER 14

Our Digital Lives: Finding Balance in the On-Demand Culture

HOW TO RUIN A GOOD CONVERSATION WITH YOUR TEEN OR YOUNG ADULT

It was about 6 PM, and I was sitting in a diner having coffee and cake with my 21-year-old. We were discussing Hans Zimmer, the music producer of the movie "12 Years a Slave," and his accomplishments. Having just been to see the movie that afternoon, we were engrossed in his website on her cell phone. We were having a great discussion.

I kept getting texts from a friend who wanted to make evening plans. Then I began getting other texts from my sister about the next day. This led to phone calls due to anticipation about bad weather. I choose to pay attention to the texts and calls and totally interrupted the dynamic discussion we were having.

After responding to the texts leading to several more phone calls, my daughter said these stinging words to me, "You are worse than me, Mom, talking on the phone in a diner, it's disgusting. My friends don't interrupt someone in mid-sentence to answer a text," she said. She was clearly feeling ignored and dismissed as I paid attention to my calls and texts. At that moment, I saw myself slip from part of the solution to part of the digital problem. Just the day before, I had fallen prey to the gripping jaws of computer and phone mania, not being able to disengage.

I replied, "You are right but wait, let's discuss this. I write and teach about these things. " I asked her what she thought might be a way for us and other families to enjoy using the phone for Wikipedia without disrupting this fun activity by answering texts and phone calls. I asked, "Is it possible to make an agreement prior to the meal to not take phone calls or texts?" We questioned whether we could implement that for ourselves and agreed to try.

It's hard as a grown up to hold back from feeling defensive when we perceive kids criticizing us for an action they do all the time. Of course it's natural to want to remind our teen or young adult of the time they texted their way through an entire meal or family gathering. Instead, a suggestion is to just take a deep breath and see this as an opening. The next time we are intending to have a conversation with our child who is texting as we speak, we can remind them that we'd like to implement these rules for the conversation.

Having an Uninterrupted Check- In Time

During high school and middle school, it helps families to have a specific in- person check- in time with teens with one or both parents present. There are some conversations where you do need the complete attention of your child, or the child wants your uninterrupted attention to share something important. Establishing a daily check-in time with your adolescent helps keep humor around stressful and important issues such as college applications, exams, homework, social, extracurricular activities and weekend plans.

Guidelines for Parents to Support a Mindful Check-In

- Establish eye contact.
- Remember to breathe.
- Request all digital devices be turned off.
- Refer to embodied communication (See Chapter 10)
- Inform the other party of time limitations.
- Agree on a time that works for parents and teen.
- Ask for a consistent time of day (such as at 7PM).
- Ask the teen to "tell me more" rather than ask why.
- Limit the conversation to 15 minutes.
- Keep it simple and direct.

Help Teens with Anxiety Transition to Homework

- Encourage the equal counting breath before beginning a task.
- Use embody cues to find the sitz bones, head to tail connection (See Chapter 6)
- Give calendar cues by looking at a calendar with parent and student to keep conscious of deadlines.
- Utilize Golden Ray, Warrior pose, and breathing to gain focus.
- Offer a visual schedule, (picture schedule of tasks) and a timer for teens with executive function issues.
- Use a simple to do list with visual cues or use an iPhone app.
- Offer yoga strategies for getting started such as Ha breath, sensory yoga feeling wheel or a guided visualization.
- Remember to breathe and practice patience and contentedness.
- Set firm boundaries in combination with small tasks so that the student experiences success in meeting the goals, e. g. , "Let's do the Warrior, Tree and the Ha breath. Then, how about you sit at the dining room table and do 10 minutes of math. I'll check back with you to see how you are doing. "

Please Park Your Phone Here

Families across the country are trying many options to limit usage of cell phones and enjoy their time with friends and family. The goal of a no cell phone gathering is to enjoy the company of others without interruption. For some kids, 30 minutes is their tolerance away from the phone. In that case, let them check their phone and respond. It isn't about a punishment, but an introduction to non-cell activity. The first few times you implement this might cause some anxiety for teens who are highly addicted to the phone or iPad.

- Provide a basket for the teens to put their cell phone in by the door.
- The goal is to be present with their friends in the here and now.
- Adults can suggest to teens to take a texting break after 30 min-60 minutes to check their texts and to then text for about 5 minutes.
- Ask the kids how long they want for the text break.
- Invite them to return to the board game, video, computer, TV, charades or talking activity that is happening with the group.
- Adults can keep providing snacks for the group to keep them interested in sustaining their activities. This also allows you to come in and enter the space and check if this is working without being too intrusive.
- The goal is about enjoying focused non-multitasked attention for the adolescents.
- Gradually you can increase the time away from the electronic usage.
- There eventually will be tolerance to stay away for hours or a day, depending on the family agreement.

What Does Your Family Like to Do That Isn't Electronic?

One approach to digital detox is to designate one day a week to completely disengage from any electronics. For this day of the week, do other activities that don't involve, phone, TV, computer, iPad, DVD etc. Or, limit most electronics and keep one only if it seems impossible to accomplish this the first time. Another variation is to do it only for the morning or the afternoon if the whole day seems too daunting at first. Activities can be a variety of sleeping, walking, talking, eating, gardening, cleaning, de-cluttering, chores, visiting some place of interest, playing a game or watching a real live game taking place in the community (not digitally).

Agree on the time that the day starts and ends and when you can get back to the electronics. The goal isn't to completely stop; it is to take a break and enjoy other things without interruption. It's perfectly fine to look forward to resuming the electronic use.

Use the day to do family and individual projects. Some examples are:

Volunteering	Gardening
Baking and Cooking	Cleaning out the garage
Playing in the town park	Visiting a book store or library
Sewing	Reading
Walking	Hiking
Biking	De-cluttering
Visiting friends or relatives	Sports, Swimming
House repairs	Washing the car
Fishing	Helping an older person
Sorting your toys or papers	Cleaning out your desk
Writing in your journal	Painting
Arts and crafts	Resting
Walking the dog	Giving the dog a bath
Cleaning out closets	Playing musical instruments
Bowling	Skateboarding

These activities are just a sampling and you can include any non-digital activity that your family enjoys. Some families may choose to make this day coincide with a day of observance, but that is not the intention. Or you may choose that there might be other particular activities that you refrain from. It is about finding some way to regain the balance you have lost from overuse of electronics. Make it a fun adventure to think up what you would like to do.

FINDING NON-DIGITAL FAMILY ACTIVITIES IN NATURE AND THE COMMUNITY

With the ever spreading overuse of technology moving into every aspect of our lives there is a loss of appreciation and participation in nature for our children. Enjoyment of outside time becomes diminished as we are more drawn to the computer for enjoyment. Unfortunately today, for many families, life's responsibilities will not easily permit time in nature; it involves a concerted effort to make outside time take place regularly. Only a short time ago, children without a phone to check for texts, or a computer game were less pressured and more able to enjoy a moment in nature or with family without distraction. Many families make great efforts to enjoy outside family time, taking a picnic, a hike, bicycling, doing a snow activity or a walk. It demands some self-discipline to set limits on the use of electronics. Yet, families and children used to be content to spend time together without electronics and enjoy a day outing. The story below reflects the way children used to enjoy time when I was growing up when the computer was not competing for our attention

A Family Day in 1961

Growing up in the 50's and 60's there were no big box stores yet. It is hard to imagine no Wal-Mart, Target, or any of the big stores that exist today. My Dad was in retail, so Sunday was his only day off. He was eager to get out of the house after lunch. Often my Dad took us on a hike in a town park, walking in mountains, skating at a pond in winter and to the town water hole in summer. There was a rhythm to the week and we knew on Sunday what to expect. We'd be going somewhere.

This is a recollection I have of a typical family day in the years before the advent of information technology at every turn. It is Sunday and we are heading into New York City and driving over the George Washington Bridge. The bridge is huge and really exciting to drive over. You can see the tall buildings and the city skyline as we cross the Hudson River. My brother and I are playing geography in the car naming a place that starts with the last letter of the word named previously. We are looking in awe at the tall bridge and at the water below. We are going to visit my aunt who has a big apartment that overlooks Central Park, a very large city park.

My aunt's apartment is filled with art and objects from her travels. She had wooden carved heads (sculptures) from Africa, bronze statues from India and beautiful dishes from Italy. She tells us many stories. She has a large glass table filling up the entire dining room, with lights inside of it, that turn on. We are sitting and having tea and biscuits. She is laughing and telling us a story. It is always fun to be with her.

We are taking a walk through Central Park with trails and paved roads. My brother and I climb the big boulders and sit on the rocks in the sun. The park has a zoo and a lake. Many people are walking in the park. It is strange to be in nature but also hear the city noises close by and see the tall buildings.

We are saying goodbye to my aunt and heading home to visit my grandmother. My grandmother greets us and takes all the children to a room in the back of her house that is always cold. She keeps homemade cookies in containers there. The cookies are always hard as a rock. She insists we have one.

Finding Non-Digital Fun Ways to Spend Time

Make a list of five things your family enjoys outdoors or indoors.

As a parent, I love nature activities because they make my senses happy, are relatively inexpensive and uplift my spirits. They are a break from the complexities of modern life, traffic and sitting. For a break from electronics, nature activities are simple, and low cost. If you are all walking together or hiking, you may want to have the phone for safety. The walking activity itself though keeps you moving and can take your mind off talking on the phone. Taking a 20 -90 minute hike all together as a family to a designated spot is an excellent activity in the city or country, can make a difference for our mind state and can be transforming energetically.

Family Nature Activities in Cities:

- Pick a street with the least amount of cars and traffic.
- Agree to a time when everyone can participate.
- Bring snacks and water, sunscreen, hat and layers, first aid.
- Check weather before setting out for safety.
- Check the trail if you are trying something new in the woods.
- Bring a map if you are in a city.
- Pick a destination to walk to.
- Avoid a mall as this won't give the nature experience.
- Determine that you aren't on someone's private property.
- Avoid hunting season in the rural areas or even outside towns.
- Hike or walk with other families for added support.
- Prepare sensory kids with extra snacks, and verbal and visual games .
- Know how long you will be hiking and when you will arrive.
- Leave a message with family or friends if going hiking.
- Have a charged cell phone in case of emergency.
- Wear adequate shoes and clothes for cold or hot (no flip flops please!)
- Do not allow teens to wear flip flops for extended walks as they can be dangerous, break along the way and cause falls.
- Wear bright colors or orange vests if you are in traffic or at dusk.

A Happy Day for Children in Nature

I was invited to my friend's son's birthday party for a 5th-6th grade class. It was a hot sunny afternoon and the party was gathering in the yard. Everyone was getting ready to take a hike in the forest along the river behind the house.

All the adults and children began a long hike through the wooded area to the riverbed. The kids picked up walking sticks and walked in groups, stopping to look at rocks and vegetation along the way. When we arrived at the edge of the riverbed we could see a long and wide expanse of dry stones that we could walk out on. There were also fallen uprooted trees from a recent storm. The kids climbed out on the limbs and sat overlooking the river. They entertained themselves for hours skipping rocks on the river. Walking along the river edge in small and large groups, they looked for the perfect smooth shaped stones and played, jumping over boulders and climbing limbs of the fallen trees.

After a while, we all gathered and started a slow walk back through the woods back to the house to get some food. Walking slowly, there was ample time for adult conversation and the kids also seemed contented and relaxed. Upon returning to the house, the girls inhabited one large seated swing. The boys took to the hammock, piling on top of one another laughing, very contented after hiking in nature and playing physically.

Going for a Non-Digital Holiday

Some families decide they need to take a complete non-digital vacation for a day outing, weekend or week leaving all the electronics at home except for an adult cell phone for emergency purposes. Whether you go to a lodge, camp, visit relatives or have a stay at home vacation, there are many variations on how to do this.

Families can go to a hotel that advertises that there are no electronics, (no TV in the room, no use of the internet) for a digital detox. They can attend a family or wilderness or faith based retreat with their family. Yoga retreats, camping with other families in the woods, camping at a lodging that provides many outside activities and cabins with other families are good options.

Set your own rules about reducing or specifying the times the electronics can be used. Often on a retreat the kids are so busy no one has any time to use the phone or iPad except for a few minutes after a meal. There may not be a need to leave the electronics at home, just be aware of the use and limits. There are also ways to enjoy outside time away and allow some digital time at night depending on how much of a detox you feel you need.

BEING MORE ACTIVE WITH TECHNOLOGY

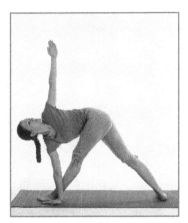

Revolved Triangle
Prep Pose

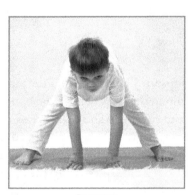

Prasaritta

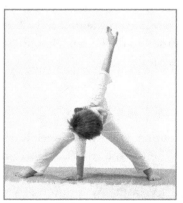

Padottanasana

Maximize Physical Activity: Use the Smart board with Yoga

- Use postures using benches or supported standing pose while facing sideways and cross midline to reach the board.
- Practice mindfulness: patience and turn-taking.
- Use a DVD to get upper body movement on the Smart board .
- Stand instead of sit.
- Assume postures before a turn at the smart board game.

Revolved Triangle Prep (Moderate-Advanced)

The Revolved Triangle illustration here needs to be adapted to use at the smart-board. In this exercise, described below, we are doing the prep for the pose with adaptations of a bench and a ball.

- Stand and face the smart board.
- Place a low bench with the long edge along the child's right side.
- Turn the body to the right, facing the long side of the bench.
- Place the left leg, or the leg closest to the smart board, up on the bench so the hips and knees are at 90 degrees or what the child is capable of. Support the child to balance and stand on the right leg.
- Hold the wand in the right hand.
- Rotating to the left, turn the torso so that the right arm holding the wand crosses midline and touches the board. For deeper rotation place the left hand directly on a surface (a secured large therapy ball) further to the left. (The right hand hits at 12 and the left is placed at 9 o'clock)

Forward Bends (Adapted *Prasaritta Padottanasana*)

- Place the bench in front of the child parallel to the smart board.
- Stand in Mountain pose.
- Give instructions to stand in a wide-legged stance.
- Similar to a forward bend, place both hands down on the bench in a modified forward bend.
- Bending forward at the hip joint, hands on the bench, weight bear into the hands, then come up halfway up, looking up.
- Reach to touch the smart board on the right or left or crossing midline

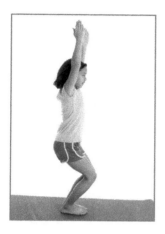

Chair Pose

Chair Pose (Revolving)(Advanced and Can Be Modified)

- Use chair pose to build core tone for more intensity.
- Stand perpendicular to the smart board with the left side closest to the board. Place a bench near the left foot (between the child and board).
- Stand in Mountain pose arms raised over the head along ears.
- Assume Chair pose as seen in illustration.
- Rotating to the left, bear weight with the right hand on a bench, surface or floor next to the left foot.
- Reach for the wand with the left hand, opening the chest, and getting rotation while twisting to tap the smart board.
- Repeat on the opposite side.

TIPS AND TAKE AWAYS

A gentle approach to changing habits of digital overuse is suggested. Just being conscious of what children are doing and holding a firm vision of what you want is helpful.

- A quiet, sweet, but firm stance is needed by parents to ask teens to put the phone away and engage in a social gathering.

- Parents need a sense of humor and perseverance to not readily give in to preschoolers' requests for iPads in restaurants.

- Clinicians can suggest to parents to pack books or crayons so children can read or color and to strategically reduce handing the phone to young children as often as they request it. The chance for embodying experiences is magnified by starting habits early.

Remember that it is perfectly acceptable, if you take a digital break, to be looking forward to a set time when you can reconvene your electronic activities. This could be at sundown or when you choose. It could be a 2-hour, a morning or afternoon break. Design what works for your family. In reducing digital use, my goal is to re-introduce the activities that the iPad is replacing. If your teen just spent several hours biking or hiking with you, playing sports, or helping with chores and you just had a quality conversation with no electronic interruption, and your teen wants to get on the computer, it appears to be a balanced approach. But if your 10-year-old has been on the computer since 8 AM and it's noon and he wants to stay home and continue instead of going out with the family on a nice day, then some boundaries need to be set and strategies put in place to create greater balance.

CHAPTER 15

The Yoga of Daily Life

REFUELING WITH BRAIN BODY TOOLS

Practicing Brain Body Tools as professionals, we can bring yoga interventions and mindfulness into the classroom and therapy sessions. As we shift more to recognize our intuition, and connect to the world around us through the body, learning is enhanced for all students. This offers new strategies for students with sensory processing issues and special needs. As parents, as we re-balance our fascination with electronics with time in nature, we can help children and ourselves to shift how we experience stress with meditation. The embodied self and mindfulness buffer us from our reactions and feelings to life's unpredictable ups and downs and facilitates the healing of trauma. As we recognize the Witness, practice embodied communication, and make time for nature, the Brain Body Tools become our re-fueling station. We now have tools to practice the yoga of daily life and take out into the world, our families and communities.

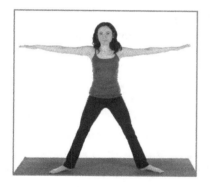

Standing Star Pose

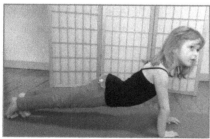

Plank Pose

Bringing Yoga Interventions into the Classroom

Standing Star and Swinging Star pose

Triangle pose

Lunge

Happy Warrior

Tree pose

Interject a yoga break in between lessons or during the transition between subjects. Alise Wright Tanny, author of *YogaPlay* (2007) pg. 43 shows how to use the Star formation for a classroom warm-up based on the basic neuro-cellular patterns from the principles of Body Mind Centering.

Swinging Star Pose

- Bending forward, bring the arms to the right leg and, pretending you will be finger painting with both hands on a pretend wall in front of you, in a circular direction, stretch out the arms to the right side to 3 o'clock position. Then, extend the arms over head to be a pointed star with arms and legs in a wide stance (2 and 10 o'clock). Bend again to the left side extending arms fully (9 o'clock) and finally down to ankles. Bend forward to center to end.
- **Standing Star** Extend arms and legs in wide stance
- **Triangle, Lunge, Tree pose,** on each side
- Silent walking for several minutes in the room
- Cross crawls and Connect-ed
- Wall pushups, Plank pose.
- Desk or chair push up
- Chair yoga twist, forward bend
- Standing backbend with hands on the desk behind you
- Cat and Cow in stand at the desk, with arms behind head
- Grounding column.

TIPS FOR CAREGIVERS: HOW TO FIT IN WALKING, YOGA OR EXERCISE DAILY

I have a dog and I try to walk 30 minutes every day in the late afternoon or evening. I find the oxygen and the exercise helps with fending off depression. The physical movement helps me to be less stiff, and it counters the computer posture and prolonged sitting from driving. But mainly the daylight and sunlight are so uplifting even in the cold.

I used to give the excuse that I had no time to walk. But after I started walking regularly, it just fit into the day and there was no loss for taking this time to myself. Instead, it serves as a bridge from the work day to the more contemplative and personal time that is my own. After the walk, I feel I can breathe easier. I can let go of the tape in my head of stressful situations that keeps replaying.

When my child was younger, I would walk with other mothers as the children rode bikes. Often, I did a yoga DVD after my child went to sleep. During some very stressful times, I would practice yoga DVD and meditation at 4:30 AM to squeeze in some movement and quiet time to keep my sanity. In different stages of parenting, opportunities for exercise can vary.

With younger children, you can just bring them with you to a square dance, for a hike, or walk with the dog. A challenging phase is when you have to drive the tweens and younger teens to so many activities, and you are left waiting in the car or on the bench. One participant from a seminar shared how she got tired of waiting outside for her daughter's yoga class. She decided to just go inside the studio and take the class with her daughter! Now they do this regularly. It has become an enjoyable bonding activity for them.

I can remember walking back and forth or around the playground during some play-dates. The mothers and I were peeled to watching the kids but determined to walk and wanted to exercise. As my daughter became older and in high school, she would do DVD's and I joined in. I had my share of waiting in the car or on the field. It took a toll evidenced by weight gain, and feeling frustrated. I finally joined the gym and got some relief, started going dancing when I could, and planned hikes and walks on weekends with friends, family or alone.

Squeeze Yoga and Exercise into Your Day

- Start the day with a Sun Salutation, 2 to 5 rounds each side.
- Keep a Thera-Band in your purse for down time.
- Use a yoga strap to stretch while watching TV.
- Plan walks as part of the day or week.
- Choose dancing, walking, bowling instead of sitting for drinks.
- Attend a yoga class regularly.
- Do 15 minutes of yoga from YouTube, DVD or follow a book.
- Schedule in cleaning house for exercise.
- Take breaks with yoga standing poses while cooking.
- Keep a set of 2-5 pound weights near your desk for break time.
- Organize chances to get up from your desk and move frequently.
- Plan yard work on weekends.

- Wake up and clean a room, or do yoga rather than check email.
- Add a seated *Vinyasa*, and twists when on Facebook®.
- Choose Warrior 2 or Triangle pose during a YouTube® video.
- Try core-building plank with the kids or when reading a book.
- Get on the floor with the kids on a regular basis.
- Declutter rather than begin the day on the computer.
- Set a time to meet the kids and walk instead of sitting in the car.
- Take part in a community 5K.
- Lift weights or do jumping jacks while watching movies.
- Commit to a yoga routine in your week.

Creating a Time for Meditation

On weekends, I get up before everyone else to tend the dog. After this, I'll bring my hot water and lemon and retreat to a special place in the house to meditate where I won't be disturbed. This makes the weekend truly delicious, because I am really giving myself this special time. Even if I can only squeeze in 10-15 minutes, that is plenty of time to go within and have a heart meditation. Create a ritual that helps you find time to do your meditation, to find a special time for yourself to contemplate and relax using the breath.

If you are a teacher or a push-in therapist who works in the classroom, what can you do to create a special contemplative time for your students? Suggestions such as sensory corners, legs up on the wall, heads on fists on the desk, the raft or balloon guided imagery, quiet time and silent meditation for a few minutes are possible activities to consider.

For therapists, what can you create within the session for a few moments that can be restful and contemplative? Refer to legs on the wall, restorative.

When in the day can you find 5-15 minutes to meditate?

Heart Meditation (See Chapter 8)

Close your eyes and focus on the heart. Allow your awareness to focus at the heart and drop into the feeling of that organ. Hold your focus there as you breathe deeply with a 4-count breath, hold for 4, exhale for 6 and hold for 2. Repeat this for several times until you feel relaxed.

Practice Pausing

We can hear the small voice of inner awareness when we take a moment to pause and sit quietly. This can help an idea or feeling come to light that we might want or need in a critical juncture or bring the pleasure and gratitude of simply being in the present moment. Instead of always moving ahead to the next thing, we can practice pausing and non-striving and be filled by what that moment brings us.

WHAT ARE WAYS YOU CAN PRACTICE PAUSING AND STAY IN THE MOMENT?

Be kind to yourself and make a practice of creating alternatives to checking your phone, iPad and email and filling your day with to do lists. Allow yourself to let yourself be, look around you and stay in the moment, listening to your own feelings and body. What happens when you do an embodied check in by focusing on breathing, shifting awareness and finding your bones and head to tail connection?

A YOGA AND FAMILY RETREAT

While raising my child, I was fortunate to participate each summer in a family retreat at my yoga foundation. No matter what your culture, faith or community, a family retreat of any kind is a special way for parents to get support. The retreat empowers children with valuable experiences, and the parents have a great time with other families. Many faith-based, athletic, arts, and community organizations have retreats for families. The following story of a day in our summer brought our family many happy memories.

It was a beautiful Friday morning in the mountains, the sun was out in a cerulean blue sky, and the children and parents were walking into the main meeting room or meditation hall. The parents and children greeted one another, happy to see new and old friends. People arrived for the weekend or weeklong retreat from near and far away places around the globe. Quickly saying our hellos, laughing and chatting, we all shared the day's excitement. There was a play of a classic tale enacted by the children happening that afternoon. All summer the children had been putting on a performance each Friday afternoon of a chapter from a classic tale. The children auditioned for the play on a Monday, learned their parts, rehearse all week and would be ready to perform on Friday. The past weeks performances had been very well done and dramatic and there was much excitement to see the newest performance later that day.

The parents settled down to sit for a short meeting and to (sing) chant with the children before dispersing to do our volunteer work gardening, preparing food, or jobs needed at the retreat. We waited for the emcee to begin. A 7- year-old girl sat in the front of the hall with the musicians, behind a harmonium (an instrument about 18 inches long and one foot wide that has a keyboard and bellows like an accordion.) Next to her was a boy the same age, sitting with a drum. Other older children sat nearby in the front. The teens would be lead chanters in the call and response song or some teens played flutes, guitars or other instruments. The hall was filled with about 80-100 children from many countries and speaking different languages. There was a special buzz in the air, and the children soon would disperse after the morning gathering to prepare for the play or chosen activities.

The emcee lightly touched the microphone to garner everyone's attention. He told the children to choose one of the morning activities, sports, nature hike, reading in the library, arts and crafts or play rehearsal. Then several children joined the stage. They performed a short story about an infamous character, Sheikh Nasrudin, who was very funny because he was so silly and foolish and everyone laughed hilariously. The story always had a teaching, and the emcee asked the children to comment on the story.

Then the musicians were signaled to start a melodic melody. Everyone joined in with a call and response song that was joyful and rhythmic. The music started out slowly then the tempo quickened and rose to a crescendo. After a short while the singing ended and everyone sat quietly for meditation, basking in the stillness within felt after singing.

I needed to get to the costume department quickly and left the hall before the morning gathering officially ended. I had to fill the costume bags for each child with all the parts of their costumes. I could hear the humming of the sewing machines, as I entered the room. Volunteers were already sewing last minute costume changes from the rehearsal the night before. The bags had to be laid out quickly as the children would soon be coming to pick them up. The kids had several costume changes and were usually multiple characters in the play. I had to focus on my task to make sure I was putting all the parts of each character's costume in the bag and not forgetting anything crucial.

Children were already coming into the costume room stressed about costumes that didn't fit and torn garments from last night's rehearsal. The room looked like chaos, but the atmosphere was filled with lots of joy. I greeted everyone and jumped into the fray of fun and excitement. The day was demanding my full attention, humor and compassion, and I was fully present.

GUIDELINES FOR A FAMILY RETREAT

The following list of guidelines can be considered when planning a retreat. Retreats may emerge from a community of like-minded individuals, a place of worship, community group or interest group. Retreats can be for a week, a weekend, an evening or a day. You can design what works for you.

I have laid out guidelines here for you to utilize if you would like to plan a retreat. Although it's fun to go away to a retreat, it is possible to plan a local retreat in your community where you live. You can have the families and children gather in a designated place during the day, but return to their homes at night. Volunteers can prepare food or everyone can brown-bag food. The important key factor is for people to enjoy the company of one another and the theme of the retreat.

Key Elements of a Family Retreat
- Retreats center on families.
- Children participate with their families (exceptions can be made for guardianship.)
- Adults do volunteer work for the retreat.
- Possibly paid staff might assist, if you are at an organized retreat center.
- Plan activities.
- Meals are taken together, children and parents.
- Music is played.
- The focus on experiential activities.

Retreat Activities

- Plays
- Arts and crafts
- Physical activities yoga, T'ai Chi,
- Dance
- Sports
- Nature walks
- Singing
- Olympics

Qualities at a Retreat

- Educational, interest-based, faith or universal teachings
- An appropriate ratio of adults to kids for safety
- Food or access to food
- Accommodations or access to
- Fun activities for the children
- Humor
- Teamwork
- Time outdoors in sports, nature
- Open and closed-eyed meditation
- Dancing
- Educational activities for adults

Suggested protocol for a retreat

1. Morning gathering: the children gather with adult leadership.

   Shares of personal experiences

   Stories with life lessons

   Singing

   Playing of musical instruments

   Special presentations showcasing children's talent

   Directions about the activities for the day

   Plays about aspects of the human condition

2. Children attend activities of their choice: arts and crafts, sports, musical instruments, nature hike, reading or weekly play.

3. Parents attend parenting groups where they can discuss challenges in parenting, have time to meditate, study, or have time to do embodying practices.

4. Community lunch and free time

5. Afternoon program

6. Dinner

7. Group Dancing

Model for a Community Meditation Group

An open group in my community meets daily for meditation at 7:30 AM. There is a short reading. A candle is lit as people enter. The group sits in a circle. The participants say "Om" 3 times in a group as they inhale and exhale, and then sit quietly for 30 minutes of silent meditation. The group leader signals the start and end of the meditation with a bell, chime or gong. After the final bell, "Om" is sung 3 times and then "Peace" is also sung 3 times with an inhale and exhale.

<u>Optional Community Activity:</u> Once a week participants are invited to meet for coffee together afterward. In this group of retired and semi-retired individuals, it evolved to going to breakfast every morning that accommodated their schedule and allowed the group to socialize. The main focus is to provide a place for meditation, and socializing is optional.

Tips and Take Aways

- Have a welcoming and accepting attitude that honors everyone.
- Come together for enjoyment and solace.
- Find a comfortable environment that is pleasant.
- Provide chairs if needed.
- Have a designated start and finish time.
- Encourage people to enter respectfully.
- Explain the agenda to new people:
  - Listen to a short reading.
  - Ring bell to start.
  - Sing "Om" 3 times.
  - Sit silently for meditation for 30 minutes.
  - Ring bell to indicate silent meditation if finished.
  - Sing "Om" 3 times.
  - Sing "Peace" 3 times.

As we practice the Brain Body Tools in this book, we are embracing a new level of self–care for ourselves and others, and taking yoga into our lives, schools and communities. Whether we are sitting for 5 minutes silently in our car and practicing an embody exercise, or watching our breath to pause before work, we are developing awareness of our intuition, the witness and tuning into our emotional state. Being silent with our morning coffee, doing a yoga intervention in the classroom to find our feet, or meditating in the mall parking lot, we start where we are at and build a commitment to cumulatively practice as we can. As we incorporate the exploration of embodied practice into our priorities, we enhance the lives of our children, clients, families, communities and ourselves.

Further Reading

Finklestein, M. (2013). 77 *Questions for skillful living: A new path to extraordinary health.* New York: Harper Collins.

Levine, P.A. & Frederick, A. (1997). *Waking the tiger: Healing trauma.* Berkeley, CA: North Atlantic Books.

Lewis, S., & Lewis, S.K. (2014). *Stress-proofing your child. Mind-body exercises to enhance your child's health.* New York: Bantam Books.

Louv, R. (2012). *The nature principle: Reconnecting with life in a virtual age.* Chapel Hill, NC: Algonquin Books.

Miller, G.W., Ethridge, P, Ethridge, M., & Tarlow, K. (2011). *Exploring body-mind centering: An anthology of experience and method.* Berkeley, CA: North Atlantic Books.

Payne, K. J. (2010). *Simplicity parenting. Using the extraordinary power of less to raise calmer, happier and more secure kids.* New York: Ballantine Books.

Van der Kolk, B. (2014). *The body keeps the score: Brain, mind and body in the healing of trauma.* New York. Penguin Books.

Flynn, L. (2013). *Yoga for children. 200 yoga poses, breathing exercises and meditations for healthier, happier, more resilient children.* Avon MA: Adams Media

RESOURCES

Residential Retreat Centers:
    Kripalu Center Stockbridge, M.A.   www.kripalu.org
    Omega Institute, Rhinebeck, N.Y.   www.eomega.org

TRAININGS

International Association of Yoga Therapists
The School for Body Mind Centering
The Yoga Center of Amherst, Massachusetts
Restorative Yoga Teachers: Judith Hanson Lasater
Life Force Yoga -Yoga for Depression
Yoga 4 Classrooms
Attunement yoga

References

Bainbridge Cohen, Bonnie. Sensing, Feeling and Action: The Experimental Anatomy of Body-Mind Centering® 2012 Northampton, Contact Editions.

Bernardi, L., Sleight, P., Bandinelli, G., Cencetti, S., Fattorinni, L., WdowczycSzulc, J., & Lagi, A.(2001). Effect of rosary prayer and yoga mantras on autonomic cardiovascular rhythms: Comparative study. -British Medical Journal,323,1446-1449.

Calhoun, Yael & Calhoun, Matthew. Create a Yoga Practice for Kids: Fun, Flexibility and Focus. 2006. Santa Fe. Sunstone Press.

Farhi, Donna. Yoga Mind, Body and Spirit: A Return to Wholeness. 2000. NY. St. Martins Press.

Gaynor L, Mitchell. Sounds of Healing: A Physician Reveals the Therapeutic Power of Sound, Voice and Music. 1999 NY. Broadway Books.

Goldberg, Louise. Yoga Therapy for Children with Autism and Special Needs. 2013 NY. Norton.

Hartley, Linda. Wisdom of the Body Moving. An Introduction to Body-Mind Centering. 1995. Berkeley. North Atlantic Books.

Kabat-Zinn, Jon. Mindfulness for Beginners: Reclaiming the present moment and your life. 2012 Boulder. Sounds True.

Kaiser Greenland, Susan. The Mindful Child: How to Help Your Kid Manage Stress and Become Happier, Kinder and More Compassionate. 2010. NY Atria.

Kaminoff, Leslie &Matthews, Amy. Yoga Anatomy: Your illustrated guide to postures, movements and breathing techniques.2012 Champaign, IL. Human Kinetics.

LaPage, Joseph & Lillian. Mudras for Healing and Transformation. 2014. Sebastopol, Ca. Integrative Yoga Therapy.

Lasater, Judith. Relax and Renew: Restful Yoga for Stressful Times. 1995. Berkeley. Rodmell.

Medina, John. Brain Rules: 12 Principles for Surviving and Thriving at work, home and School. 2014. Seattle Washington. Pear Press.

Miller, Lucy Jane. Sensational Kids: Hope and Help for Children with Sensory Processing Disorder. 2006. NY. Perigree.

Naparstek, Belleruth. Invisible Heroes: Survivors of Trauma and How They Heal. 2004. New York. Bantam.

Olsen, Andrea. BODYSTORIES: A Guide to Experiential Anatomy.1998. Lebanon, NH. University Press of New England.

Siegel, Daniel J. The Mindful Brain: Reflection and Attunement in the Cultivation of Well Being. 2007.New York: W.W. Norton & Company.

Weintraub, Amy. Yoga Skills for Therapists: Effective Practices for Mood Management. 2012.NY. Norton.

Wood Valley, Sarah. Sensational Meditation for Children: Mindful Guided Imagery and Other Child-Friendly Meditation Techniques. 2013. Asheville, NC . Satya Worldwide

Wright-Tanny, Alisa. YogaPlay: A Mind body Centering Approach. 2007 Northampton. Paradise Copies.

Study- Kaiser Foundation.

Generation M2: Media in the Lives of 8- to 18-Year-Olds. Jan 2010. Henry J. Kaiser Family Foundation. Menlo Park Ca.